T0271005

Human Guinea Pigs

First published in 1967, *Human Guinea Pigs* is a report by a consultant physician on the implications of medical research on both the medical profession and on the men, women and children who are the subjects of medical experiments. It suggests that there are limits to the permissibility of experiments on humans. It points out how it has become a common occurrence for medical investigators to take risks with patients of which the patients themselves are frequently unaware, and to submit them to mental and physical distress and possible hazards which in no way are necessitated by or have connection with the treatment of the disease from which are suffering. The author describes a number of experiments which, in his opinion, raise important problems. In his view, medical research must go on, but there *must* be acknowledged and observed safeguards for patients. This book will be of interest to students of medicine, ethics, law, politics and social work.

Human Guinea Pigs

Experimentation on Man

M. H. Pappworth

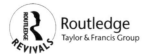

Routledge
Taylor & Francis Group

First published in 1967
By Routledge & Kegan Paul

This edition first published in 2022 by Routledge
4 Park Square, Milton Park, Abingdon, Oxon, OX14 4RN
and by Routledge
605 Third Avenue, New York, NY 10017

Routledge is an imprint of the Taylor & Francis Group, an informa business

Publisher's Note
The publisher has gone to great lengths to ensure the quality of this reprint but points out that some imperfections in the original copies may be apparent.

Disclaimer
The publisher has made every effort to trace copyright holders and welcomes correspondence from those they have been unable to contact.

A Library of Congress record exists under LCCN: 67096481

ISBN: 978-1-032-44225-9 (hbk)
ISBN: 978-1-003-37118-2 (ebk)
ISBN: 978-1-032-44245-7 (pbk)

Book DOI 10.4324/9781003371182

HUMAN GUINEA PIGS

Experimentation on Man

M. H. PAPPWORTH

LONDON

ROUTLEDGE & KEGAN PAUL

*First published in 1967
by Routledge & Kegan Paul Limited
Broadway House, 68–74 Carter Lane
London, E.C.4*

*Printed in Great Britain
by W. & J. Mackay & Co. Ltd.
Chatham*

© *M. H. Pappworth 1967*

This book is dedicated to my four sources of inspiration, my wife Jean (Ayshet Chayil – 'a woman of worth') and Joanna, Dinah and Sara, our delightful daughters

CONTENTS

PREFACE

The main purpose of this book is to show that the ethical problems arising from human experimentation have become one of the cardinal issues of our time. That this is so, I hope no reader will doubt after completion of this book. I believe that only by frank discussion among informed people, lay as well as medical, can a solution be reached. The hope is that by presenting the facts in a dispassionate way this book will stimulate both the lay public and their doctors to seek a solution.

The vast majority of the medical profession are either genuinely ignorant of the immensity and the complexity of the problem or wish purposely to ignore the whole matter by sweeping it under the carpet. Even fewer lay people have any conception of the issues involved. But the medical profession must no longer be allowed to ignore the problems or to assert, as they so often do, that this is a matter to be solved by doctors themselves. The position has been well stated by a non-medical.

> Modern medicine has provoked some serious moral questions, not through malignant perversity, but because of the enormous momentum medical science has gained in the past few decades. . . .
>
> There is the nagging question, What are the permissible limits and the proper conditions for experimentation on human beings? . . .
>
> These decisions cannot be postponed indefinitely. It is crucial at this historic juncture that the enormity of the problem of discovering clear moral insights to delineate some acceptable boundaries and limits to the use of human beings in research, should not produce either an impatience or moral cyncism.[1]

During private discussion of this subject I have frequently been attacked by doctors who contend that by such publication

[1] S. E. Stumpf, of Department of Philosophy, Vanderbilt University, Nashville, Tennessee, *Annals of Internal Medicine*, 1966, **64**, 460.

Preface

I am doing a great disservice to my profession, and, more especially, that I am undermining the faith and trust that lay people have in doctors. For a long time there have been rumours that I intended to publish this book and, as a result, I have been subjected to frequent telephone calls, almost entirely from strangers, in an attempt to persuade me to abandon the project.

Other doctors and lay people have attempted to persuade me that the wiser course would be to continue to attempt to publish my views in medical journals and so avoid completely any discussion outside professional circles. An important fact is that those journals which publish accounts of the worst types of experiments do not have correspondence columns. When I have spoken on this subject of human experimentation to medical societies, the usual reaction has been, 'This does not concern us, as we do not do such things', and the problems posed are ignored. Mundane, material matters of pay, status and terms of service would, in contrast, produce a lively discussion.

I am fully aware of the fact that lay people may find the accounts of some of the experiments difficult to follow, indeed the complexity of many of them is such that it is difficult even for many doctors to understand everything. So I do not expect lay people to do so, but hope that the general gist of what the experiments involve will be obtained from these necessarily brief summaries. The diagrams of the circulation drawn by my wife should be consulted frequently.

Some readers may find that much appears to be repetitious. This has been done purposely in an attempt to convey a true picture of medical research, which indeed is frequently repetitious, almost identical experiments being performed time and time again by different research workers. This is partly due to the maniacal impulse which dominates the medical world today to publish research papers, promotion and subsequent success often depending on it. But original ideas are rare, and the adage, 'To be original you must not read – it has all been described before', is very true when applied to medical research. The apparently repetitious accounts in this volume serve to emphasize that most of the examples quoted are not isolated unusual instances but fairly common practice.

Preface

I am in full agreement with an American lawyer who said:

I wish to suggest that there are limits to the permissibility of experimentation . . . and that they require more attention and respect than lawyers, ethicists or experimental scientists have been giving them.[1]

The degree to which anti-humanism dominates modern medicine can be judged by the significant fact that in most medical reports of patients having been submitted to experimentation, the patients themselves are collectively described as 'the material'.

The author is greatly indebted to Mr. Stuart Smith for his considerable help in preparation of the manuscript, and to his wife, Jean, for the proof-reading.

[1] E. Cahn, Professor of Law, New York University of Law, *New York University Law Review*, 1961, **38,** 1.

'May I never see in the patient anything but a fellow creature in pain.'

Moses Maimonides (twelfth-century Rabbi and physician)

INTRODUCTION

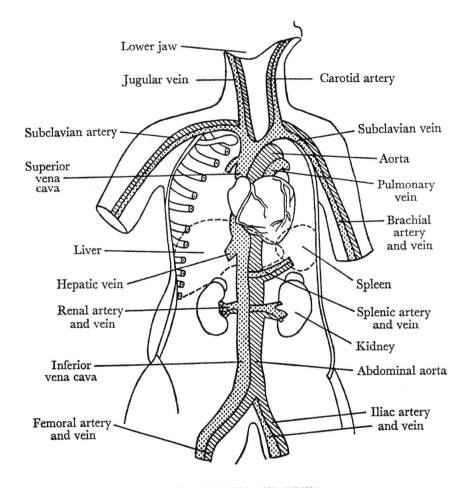

Lower jaw

Jugular vein — Carotid artery

Subclavian artery — Subclavian vein

Superior vena cava — Aorta

Pulmonary vein

Brachial artery and vein

Liver — Spleen

Hepatic vein — Splenic artery and vein

Renal artery and vein — Kidney

Inferior vena cava — Abdominal aorta

Iliac artery and vein

Femoral artery and vein

MAIN ARTERIES AND VEINS

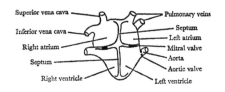

Superior vena cava — Pulmonary veins

Inferior vena cava — Septum

Right atrium — Left atrium

Mitral valve

Septum — Aorta

Aortic valve

Right ventricle — Left ventricle

CHAMBERS OF THE HEART

For several years a few doctors in this country and in America have been trying to bring to the attention of their fellows a disturbing aspect of what have become common practices in medical research. These practices concern experiments made chiefly on hospital patients and the aspect of them which is disturbing is the ethical one. In their zeal to extend the frontiers of medical knowledge, many clinicians appear temporarily to have lost sight of the fact that the subjects of their experiments are in all cases individuals with common rights and in most cases sick people hoping to be cured. As a result it has become a common occurrence for the investigator to take risks with patients of which those patients are not fully aware, or not aware at all, and to which they would not consent if they were aware; to subject them to mental and physical distress which is in no way necessitated by, and has no connexion with, the treatment of the disease from which they are suffering; and in some cases deliberately to retard the recovery from that disease so that investigation of a particular condition can be extended.

Little heed has been paid by the experimenters themselves to the occasional voices raised in protest against these practices, and there has been, on the part of editors of professional journals, some censorship of the expression of the protest – presumably from fear of offending some of their readers. Thus the editor of *The Lancet*, when refusing to publish a letter of mine on this subject some years ago, wrote me that,

> I know there are times when good comes of speaking strongly and by giving maximum publicity to what appear to be public scandals: but you haven't yet persuaded us here that this is one one of those occasions.

And an editorial in the *World Medical Journal* reveals a similar circumspection when, in commenting on the procedures used by some experimenters, it says, 'There are undoubtedly some who have failed to resist an inclination for morbid curiosity[1] –

[1] *World Medical Journal*, 1955, **2**, 21.

and leaves the matter there. While the *British Medical Journal*, though going considerably further, is still understating matters:

> There has been for some time public uneasiness about investigations carried out in hospitals which have not always been obviously in the interests of the subject of the investigations. . . .
> We could add other examples, including those given by Dr. Pappworth,[1] to indicate that the physician's human obligations to his patients are sometimes abused. . . . Undoubtedly, many investigations have been done which have been harmful to patients, even if only temporarily. And probably too many pointless investigations have been made.[2]

The truth is that many investigations have been performed which have been harmful to many patients. How temporary that harm has been is usually not known. But sometimes it definitely has not been temporary, and sometimes it has been fatal.

Any valid approximation of just how frequently medical experimentation occurs cannot possibly be given. What an American sociologist has written about America, I think is also an accurate picture of Britain.

> Precise statistics regarding the amount of human experimentation which is being conducted in present-day American medicine are hard to obtain. However, the general concensus on the part of persons currently writing about this form of medical research seems to be that in recent years the felt need for such experimentation on human subjects and its actual occurrence in our society have dramatically increased.[3]

That some risk or some distress to the subject, which is quite unrelated to the treatment of his disease is a frequent concomitant of medical experiments is indicated, or suggested, by the fact that in Britain at least, such experiments are never carried out on private patients. They are reserved for what is known as the 'hospital class'.

The subject of this book is the relation between what is morally right and what is performed in medical experiments.

---

[1] *Twentieth Century*, Autumn 1962.

[2] Editorial, *British Medical Journal*, 1962, **2, 118.**

[3] R. C. Fox, Associate Professor of Sociology, Columbia University, N.Y., *Clinical Pharmacology and Therapeutics*, 1960, **1,** 423.

The Subject

My purpose in writing it is to enlighten the public about what is going on in such experiments; to stir the consciences of the doctors so engaged and to ask them to reflect on some of the ancillary results of what they are doing and the moral issues involved. I shall also try to indicate the principles on which medical experiments should be carried out, so that the ends of research may be effectively served without any of the harm done at present, and to suggest possible legislative changes and changes in accepted procedure in which these principles may be incorporated.

This book is accordingly divided into two sections. The first of these describes a number of experiments which have been carried out in recent years. The second attempts to state the principles which should apply to such experiments and to suggest possible legislative and procedural changes in which these principles could be embodied.

The instances which I shall cite range over more than twenty years and several countries, but they refer, in the main, to what has occurred in the last ten years and, almost exclusively, in Britain and America. In Britain they are drawn chiefly, but not entirely, from teaching hospitals. It must be emphasized that whilst the vast majority of patients in hospitals are not subjected to experimentation, the number who are is considerable, although exact figures cannot be known.

The number of medical journals published is enormous. The Royal Society of Medicine of London obtains annually 2,300 differently titled current medical journals, *The Lancet*, which is published weekly, counting as one title. Indeed, it has been estimated that over 6,000 medical journals are now published in the world annually. Obviously the percentage of these which I personally have read is very small, and thus the number of experiments on human beings which I personally have read about may also be but a small fraction of the total. Moreover, those which are described in this book represent only a selection of the material known to me. It must also be emphasized that many experiments are never reported in medical journals, and I have good grounds for believing that they are often the worst of all.

Let me try to put the matter in perspective. If you, reader, were admitted to a non-teaching hospital for a comparatively minor illness such as haemorrhoids, a rupture, a broken leg, bronchitis or indigestion, there is only a very small chance, at least in Britain, of any of the kind of experiments described in this book being carried out on you. But if the hospital were a teaching or associated one, that remote chance becomes a distinct possibility although not a probability. If you have some more serious disease, especially of the heart, lungs, liver or kidneys, the same applies, but then any research undertaken is likely to be directly related to the condition from which you suffer. If your illness is not one of these, the connexion between any experiment and your particular condition is likely to be nil.

A summary of my views on medical experimentation was contained in a letter to the *British Medical Journal* in 1963[1] as follows:

(1) Clinical research must go on, but there must be acknowledged and observed safeguards for the patients. At present such safeguards are virtually non-existent.

(2) The majority of those engaged in clinical research act with the highest moral integrity, but an expanding minority resort to unethical and probably illegal practices.

(3) Unless the medical profession itself stops the unethical practices of this minority, the public outcry will eventually be such as to cause opposition to all clinical research.

Until now the profession has made no serious attempt to intervene.

The comparatively few doctors who, though they themselves do not engage in human experiments, know the facts about these activities, are either completely unwilling to discuss the subject, especially when approached by lay people, or pooh-pooh the whole matter.

At a Patients' Association meeting held in May 1965 a questioner asked about the use of patients in medical experiments without their knowledge or consent. To this Professor K. Hill, pathologist to Royal Free Hospital, London, replied[2] that this was an emotionally loaded question, which conjured up pictures of white-coated, blood-handed doctors standing over

[1] *British Medical Journal*, 1963, **2**, 505.
[2] Reported in *Medical News*, 14 May 1965.

dying dogs; or of wartime Nazi experimenters. It was most important to realize that in the long run the only way to improve medicine was to experiment, but that such experiments were rigorously controlled, and were all for the ultimate benefit of patients themselves. It was too easy to exaggerate the misdemeanours of the one or two black sheep, which any big profession must contain, who hit the headlines. I wish that Professor Hill had told his audience how experiments on patients are rigorously controlled. Although I have been interested in the subject for many years, I am completely ignorant of any such rigorous controls.

Concerning human experimentation, the desirable relationship between the medical profession and the lay public has been admirably put by a distinguished American lawyer:

> It behoves the medical profession to take the public into its confidence. The primary step is to recognize that difficult moral problems – indeed the moral dilemma – do exist of which help and guidance can be sought from many sources. In the end we have to accept the fact that some limits do exist to the search for knowledge.[1]

Although a number of doctors have voiced their concern at the way in which medical experiments have been and are being carried out, I should stress the very important fact that few doctors, and this is particularly the case with general practitioners, are fully aware of what really happens especially in many teaching hospitals, to the patients whom they send to those hospitals. This I know from discussion with hundreds of doctors over the years. A large percentage of doctors who are themselves studying to be consultants, and who are not themselves engaged in the type of research which I have written about here, are also unaware of what is going on. Many conversations with postgraduates have convinced me of this. Nor is discussion about research experiments encouraged, in their fellow doctors, by those in charge of research. Rather the reverse. It is a recent and growing practice for some research workers to work behind closed doors, which not even their own junior medical staff are encouraged to enter.

[1] Professor F. A. Freund, of Harvard Law School, *New England Journal of Medicine*, 1965, **273**, 687.

Introduction

2. RECENT HISTORY

What constitutes an experiment: physician-friend and physician-investigator

During the last twenty years clinical medicine,[1] especially in the teaching hospitals, has become dominated by research workers whose primary interest is the extension of medical knowledge. Their concern with patients as such, that is, as individual people who are sick, has tended to suffer as a result. As a distinguished Guy's surgeon, Sir William Heneage Ogilvie, has written:

> The science of experimental medicine is something new and sinister; for it is capable of destroying in our minds the old faith that we, the doctors, are the servants of the patients whom we have undertaken to care for, and, in the minds of the patients, the complete trust that they can place their lives or the lives of their loved ones in our care.[2]

The need to abide, in medical research, by the values implied in Sir William Heneage Ogilvie's statement is expressed clearly and emphatically by a distinguished American doctor, Dr. S. S. Ketty, who has for many years been engaged in research:

> The moral obligation to perform all human experiments only after due regard to the sensibility, welfare and safety of the subject must never be violated.[3]

That the danger against which Sir William Heneage Ogilvie warns and the moral obligation of which Dr. Ketty speaks have alike been widely disregarded is very clear from what has been reported in medical journals. Articles by individual research workers and by leaders of teams engaged on research reveal the

---

[1] 'Clinical' medicine is essentially bedside medicine and characteristically includes the taking of a patient's history and examining him by conventional methods. Neither the radiologist nor the pathologist, both of whose work may be essential for diagnosis, are clinicians. They are 'back-room boys' dealing with particular aspects of 'a case' and not with a patient as a whole human being. Clinical medicine is also distinct from that aspect of medicine which deals with the health and sickness of a social group – which is the sphere of Public Health.

[2] *Lancet*, 1952, **2**, 820.

[3] Quoted by H. K. Beecher in his book, *Experimentation in Man* (Charles Thomas, 1959).

frequency with which extremely unpleasant and often dangerous experiments are performed on unsuspecting patients. Most
of those doctors who know that these things are common
practice have felt powerless to stop them; while the public, for
its part, has remained unaware of what is going on.

Some apologists for the kind of experiment I shall describe
have quibbled about the meaning of the word 'experiment'.
Their argument has been that every administration of medicine
to a patient and every routine radiological or biochemical
investigation is an experiment; that, therefore, experiment is
inseparable from medicine; and that therefore any kind of
experiment by any doctor is intrinsically justified. On this basis
the empirical giving of an antibiotic to see if it will abate a high
fever, or the performance of a barium X-ray to determine
whether a patient's dyspepsia is due to a pepetic ulcer are experiments. So, in one sense, they are. But the experiments with
which I am concerned cannot, by any stretch of the imagination,
be deemed analogous. The first (such as administering an antibiotic in the case of a high fever) are directed solely to the
treatment and cure of that one patient to whom they are
administered; the second are directed, solely in some cases and
chiefly in all cases, to the discovery of what may help other
patients. Dr. Beecher, in *Experimentation in Man*, and in a passage
where he emphasizes the importance of the patient's consent,
has explained this difference clearly.

> Every act of a doctor designed soundly to relieve or cure a given
> patient is experimentation of an easily justifiable kind. The
> patient's placement of himself in the doctor's hands is evidence
> of consent. The problem becomes a knotty one when the acts
> of the physician are directed not toward the benefit of the
> patient present but towards patients in general. Such action
> requires the explicit consent of the *informed* patient. It also re-
> quires more than this; it requires profound thought and con-
> sideration on the part of the physician, for the complexities of
> medicine are in some cases so great it is not reasonable to
> expect that the patient can be adequately informed as to the
> full implications of what his consent means. His trust in the
> physician may lead him too easily to say 'yes'.

For the purpose of this book I shall regard a medical experiment as a procedure which falls within the definition laid down

9

Introduction

by Professor McCance, Professor of Experimental Medicine at Cambridge:

> We should, I think, for present purposes, regard anything done to the patient which is not generally accepted as being for his direct therapeutic benefit or as contributing to the diagnosis of his disease, as constituting an experiment, and falling therefore within the scope of the term experimental medicine.[1]

A report on human experimentation submitted to the Netherlands Minister of Health in 1955 defined it as, 'Intervention in the psychic and/or somatic integrity of man which exceeds in nature or extent those in common practice. Such an intervention may be an act either of commission or omission.'[2]

Dr. Guttentag, of the University Medical School, California, in his excellent review of the subject, wrote:

> ... experiments on the sick which are of no immediate value to them but which are made to confirm or dispute some doubtful or suggestive biological generalization. Recently this type of experiment has become more and more extensive.[3]

As I have already asserted, the teaching hospitals have tended to become dominated by doctors whose main, and even sometimes whose only, interest is research. In some cases these doctors have become so intent on achieving scientific and technical advances that they have never developed the art of taking patients' histories properly. They have come to despise ordinary clinical examination of patients by the established means of using their eyes and hands and such simple instruments as thermometer, torch, watch, stethoscope, sphygmomanometer (for blood pressure) and reflex hammer. In some cases the desire to achieve the ends of research has even caused those in its thrall to despise – or to seem to despise – that side of medicine, which is its primary side, which concerns the treatment of the patient himself. The view that the ends of research and those of therapeutic medicine as generally understood are not only different, but actually opposed, has been put forcibly by the famous Hungarian research physician, now resident in

[1] Presidential Address to the Royal Society of Medicine, *Proceedings of Royal Society of Medicine*, 1951, **44**, 189.
[2] Quoted in *World Medical Journal*, 1957, **4**, 299.
[3] *Science*, 1953, **117**, 207.

Boston, U.S.A., Dr. Szent-Gyorgi, who clearly sees the first as the great business of medicine and the second as something of much less importance. Speaking in 1961 at an international medical congress, he said:

> The desire to alleviate suffering is of small value in research – such a person should be advised to work for a charity. Research wants egotists, damned egotists, who seek their own pleasure and satisfaction, but find it in solving the puzzles of nature.[1]

Undoubtedly there are a number of British and American doctors who would privately agree with Dr. Szent-Gyorgi and would regard the following description, by Dr. Guttentag, of the relationship between what he calls the 'physician-friend' and the patient (and which occurs in the article already quoted), as a piece of sentimentality.

> One human being is in distress, in need, crying for help; and another human being is concerned and wants to assist him. The cry for help and the desire to render it precipitate their relationship. Theirs is the relationship between two I's, like between lovers, friends, pupil and teacher. I have called such a relationship 'the mutual obligation of two equals'.

To this concept of what he calls the physician-friend, Dr. Guttentag contrasts what he calls the physician-investigator.

> The physician-patient relationship of one who performs experiments of no immediate value to the person under observation is impersonal and objective because of the character of the research. Experimentation is the only basis on which they meet. But even though he is the subject in the grammatical sense, he is not the subject in the real personal sense. Every effort is made to depersonalize him and to eliminate every subjective factor. Invoked by the drive for generalization and specialization, objectivity is the password throughout.

And Dr. Bean, of Iowa, in his presidential address to the Society of Clinical Research in Chicago in 1952, drew a similar distinction:

> The danger is that the most praiseworthy zeal for knowledge may lead the man whose technical background overshadows

[1] *Lancet*, 1961, **1**, 1394.

his caring for the patients into a disregard for the subject of his researches. Thus potentially dangerous experiments may be done without the subject's knowledge or express permission. Whether it be thoughtlessness or heartlessness, such practice is a measure of the moral obliquity which exists in some high places in research today . . . Clinical investigators rarely meditate on the wide cleavage which separates clinicians from investigators in their split personality. As physicians their prime concern is the intimate personal responsibility in caring for sick people. As investigators they are goaded by discontent and impelled by curiosity as well as ambition for renown. Such stimuli sometimes suppress the physician altogether.[1]

We can contrast the physician who *accepts* patients and is always primarily concerned with their welfare, recognizing 'a mutual obligation of two equals' and the research worker who *selects* subjects (problems as well as individuals) and whilst not completely ignoring the patient's interests is mainly concerned with solving a scientific problem.

3. THE RISK TO PATIENTS

With but few exceptions, all experiments are a voyage into the unknown, and thus they must carry some risk of the untoward happening. The informed patient who accepts that risk is gambling, but an important feature of that gamble is that the patient has *personally* something worth while to gain if the experiment is directly concerned with the relief of his symptoms. But the position is entirely altered if there is no likelihood of the patient himself benefiting. As a Professor of Medicine has set out so clearly:

A much more difficult set of problems is presented in studies which involve patients or healthy subjects in experiments wherein the individual *per se* has no reasonable chance for gain aside from the satisfaction that may be derived from a sense of service to society, or more mundane gains in the form of reimbursement in cash, or, in the case of prisoners, the possibility of reward in the form of privileges or parole. There is no serious doubt that experiments of this category on humans are important if we are to advance our information and under-

---

[1] *Journal of Laboratory and Clinical Medicine*, 1952, **39**, 3.

standing of physiology, pathology, disease prevention, cure, or amelioration. Nevertheless in each case the person involved is subjected to a risk. Furthermore, the risk is not even a good gamble, since the subject has nothing to gain except perhaps money or some other value mentioned a moment ago.[1]

An often-repeated defence of the types of experiment described in subsequent chapters is that the risk of death is very small and that any complications which occur do so rarely and are generally 'trivial', and that the experiments sound much more gruesome than they really are. How gruesome an experiment may be, in fact, depends, among other things, on the emotional make-up of its subject. What may appear relatively innocuous to the hardened experimenter can produce extreme distress, including a good deal of fear, in a patient who is being submitted to something he does not understand properly. Usually he does not understand it at all. Such distress, endured by the subjects of experiments, is rarely recorded in medical publications and often appears to be of small concern to the experimenters who have caused it.

For example, if a needle inserted into a patient during the course of an experiment accidentally penetrates, say, his spleen, kidney or liver and causes a massive haemorrhage, the result will be severe physical and mental distress to that patient. In particular this will be the case if the patient realizes that something has gone wrong. However, the experimenter is likely to record it as a trivial incident immediately corrected by blood transfusion.

A typical example is a report[2] of a new method of passing a catheter[3] against the blood stream via a branch of the femoral artery of the thigh into the aorta itself, as it arises from the heart. (See diagram p. 2.) The catheter was also passed into the right or left main renal artery. A contrast medium[4] was

[1] L. G. Welt, Professor of Medicine, North Carolina University, N.C., *Connecticut Medicine*, 1961, **25**, 75.

[2] W. E. Goodwin, Scardino and W. W. Scott, of Johns Hopkins Hospital, Baltimore, *Annals Surgery*, 1950, **132**, 944.

[3] A catheter is a long thin hollow tube of plastic or rubber. A cardiac catheter is one which is passed along a vein or artery of a limb until it enters the heart. Sometimes it is passed through the heart into a more remote artery or vein.

[4] A contrast medium is a substance used by a radiologist in order to show up the organ or blood-vessels he is photographing on X-ray films.

Introduction

then injected through the catheter and serial X-rays taken. This was done on fourteen patients whilst under a general anaesthetic. The authors state, 'There have been no serious complaints. However, there have been several troublesome mishaps, which may be attributed to the method, but which are more likely to be related to the fact that it was a new technic.'

But the report records that one patient developed enlarged glands in his groin; another had breakdown of the wound over the femoral artery; two had temporary numbness over the thigh; two had moderately severe haemorrhage at the time of the catheterization; and one complained of residual weakness of his thigh muscles, which had not completely cleared two months later. Moreover, one of the patients had previously had a leg amputated because of gangrene produced by the arterial disease known as thrombo-angitis obliterans. On attempting to pass the catheter through the femoral artery of his remaining leg, the authors inform us 'unfortunately ill-advised force was used'. As a consequence a hole was made in the artery, but luckily no serious damage resulted. One of the patients submitted to this experimental procedure was aged eighty.

Or, consider the more complex technique of radiological visualization of the coronary arteries (coronary angiography). In order to obtain more satisfactory X-ray pictures some experimenters deliberately induce stoppage of the heart (cardiac arrest). One group has achieved this by passing a catheter against the blood stream via a main limb artery, into the thoracic aorta as it arises from the heart. (See diagram[1].) A balloon is attached to the end of the catheter and this is inflated until it obstructs the circulation in the thoracic aorta, the main artery arising from the heart. As a result of this procedure the heart is brought to a standstill, and then the contrast medium is injected. Two leading experts on coronary angiography have written of this technique:[2]

> The combined hazards of sudden obstruction to left ventricular outflow and accidental displacement of the balloon made routine use seem undesirable.

[1] Dotter and Frische, Oregon Medical School, Portland, Oregon, *Radiology*, 1958, **71**, 502.
[2] F. Mason Sones, Jr., and Earl Shirey, of Cleveland Clinic, Ohio, *Modern Concepts of Cardiovascular Diseases*, 1962, **31**, 735.

The Risk to Patients

Another group of physicians described a technique for producing cardiac arrest in the course of coronary angiography by the injection of a powerful drug, acetylcholine, via the catheter, directly into the heart.[1] Their first report was of having done this on twenty-three patients with coronary artery disease, the period of cardiac arrest lasting from two to thirty-two seconds. The authors wrote of their own technique:

> It may well become the method of choice for coronary angiography if the dangers of cardiac arrest are not too prohibitive.

Since then this procedure of producing heart stoppage by acetylcholine prior to the injection of the contrast medium into the coronary arteries has been performed on many patients. However, the American experts previously quoted said of the method,[2]

> This seemed undesirable because of the variable response of different patients to similar doses of the drug, and because we feared the consequences of its use in patients with unknown degrees of myocardial ischaemia [the result of coronary disease].

More recently, a British cardiologist wrote of the technique,[3] 'We never dared apply this to human subjects.'

American experts developed a new technique of coronary angiography.[4] This consists of making an opening into a main artery of an upper limb, and passing a wire guide and catheter through this hole, and, under X-ray control, along the arteries until the catheter enters the aorta and then, in turn, the orifices of the right and left coronary arteries, which are branches of the aorta itself. A contrast medium is injected directly into each coronary artery and serial cine X-rays are taken.

In a personal letter to me, dated 13/2/64, one of these heart specialists informed me that he had done over 2,500 coronary angiographies by this method within a three-year period. There

[1] Stauffer Lehman, R. A. Boyer and F. S. White, of Hahneman Hospital, Philadelphia, Pa., *American Journal Roentgenology*, 1959, **81**, 749.

[2] F. Mason Sones, Jr., and Earl Shirey, of Cleveland Clinic, Ohio, *Modern Concepts of Cardiovascular Diseases*, 1962, **31**, 735.

[3] A. Leatham, of St. George's Hospital, London, *Cardiologia* (Switzerland), 1966, **480**, 290.

[4] Sones and Shirey, ibid.

were four deaths due to the procedure. But in no less than forty-five patients the grave heart irregularity known as ventricular fibrillation occurred. Until the introduction of treatment by powerful electrical shock to the heart (defibrillator) this condition was invariably fatal. But concerning it the authors have written,

> Incidentally, in all these instances when ventricular fibrillation occurred it was possible to continue the procedure after effective counter-shock, and to complete the original objectives.

Does the fact that a new treatment has been recently discovered which is usually successful, of the very serious condition ventricular fibrillation, justify the view that the accidental production of this condition is of little consequence? Certainly, the patients themselves will not know that they have been so near to death (and the same applies to the deliberate production of cardiac arrest), although sometimes a large burn on the chest, produced by the high-voltage electrical shock which has been applied to stimulate the heart back to normal rhythm, will be evidence of that dramatic episode. Moreover, in their report the authors wrote:

> Segmental occlusion at the site of the brachial arteriotomy has occurred in 6 to 7% of the patients [as a result of the angiography]. Collateral circulation has been adequate in all of these to prevent tissue loss. A few of the group have complained of claudication (pain on movement] and sensitivity to cold, but the majority are asymptomatic three months after the procedure.

Put into lay terms, as a result of an incision made into the brachial artery so as to pass the catheter, the artery sometimes becomes blocked, thereby interfering with the blood supply of the hand. But we are led to believe that this is of little consequence. It is of interest that one of these experts on coronary angiography has expressed the opinion that heads of government, business executives and air pilots should submit to periodic coronary angiography.[1]

A group of doctors[2] reported that they have done coronary

[1] *Medical News*, 10 July 1964.
[2] Stauffer Lehman, P. Novack, Hratch Kasparian, Likoff and Perlmutter, of Hahnemann Hospital, Philadelphia, Pa., *Radiology*, 1964, **83,** 846.

angiographies by the same technique as just described (page 15) on a hundred and five patients with heart disease, varying in age from twelve to sixty-nine. There was one death as a direct result of the procedure. Another patient developed the extremely serious abnormal heart rhythm designated ventricular fibrillation, but this responded to external electrical stimulation to the chest. Two other patients developed cardiac arrest for twenty-five and twenty-seven seconds respectively, which was associated with syncope, but recovered spontaneously. In all these three instances the procedure was continued to final completion in spite of the dramatic events. In another patient the coronary artery was accidentally perforated, with the result that the contrast medium was injected into the heart muscle. This patient experienced as a consequence severe chest pain and a marked fall of blood pressure. But we are assured that within seventy-two hours the patient had made a complete recovery.

An electrocardiograph nearly always showed changes of a transitory nature, but none the less identical with those seen in coronary thrombosis. Such electrocardiograph changes are very common in any method of coronary angiography at the time of injection of the contrast medium, but their transient nature is regarded by experimenters as proof of their insignificance. I am far from convinced that this can be wholly acceptable or dismissed so casually.

As a result of the investigation four patients had an apparently permanent absence of the radial pulse due to blockage of the radial or brachial artery. Concerning this complication (discussed previously) the authors comment:

> With others, we have some apprehension as to possible serious sequelae from narrowing of the brachial artery lumen at the site of arteriotomy (incision in the artery). We believe that if the arteriotomy and its repair are meticulously performed, serious arterial insufficiency can be kept to such a minimum that it does not present a material impediment to the procedure.

Coronary angiography is an example of a lack of clear distinction between what is experimental and what is necessary for proper diagnosis and treatment. The procedure has been used extensively in a few American heart clinics. The reasons usually given for this investigation include: (1) Localization

17

and assessment of the extent of the disease in patients with known coronary artery disease with a possible consideration for surgery. (2) A desirable investigation in patients with aortic valve disease, especially if they have heart pain and if surgery of the aortic valve is contemplated. (3) The elucidation of the cause of obscure chest pain. (4) An attempt to explain why symptomless patients are found to have an abnormal tracing on a routine electrocardiography. (5) A 'routine investigation' even in the absence of any suspicion of the presence of coronary artery disease, in order to exclude its presence. (6) An attempt to further our understanding of coronary disease.

In most published series dealing with coronary angiography the actual number of patients for whom surgery has been seriously contemplated must have been very few. Certainly the patients should be informed of the high mortality rate and poor results of such surgery. They are not entirely due to its novelty, but stem in a large measure from the way the disease develops. It is very rarely localized to a small portion of a coronary artery, but is usually very extensive and therefore not amenable to local excision of one diseased portion of the artery. Furthermore, many apparently successful operations have been recorded which were followed a few months later by further attacks of coronary thrombosis.

A group of British doctors, accepting only the first three indications for this investigation of the six previously listed, found only twenty-six suitable cases in the three-year period 1963–5. Ten of these patients had chronic coronary artery disease, but only two were deemed suitable for surgery. Unfortunately, both of these patients died immediately after the operation, although seven of the others in the same group who were not submitted to surgery were still alive three years later.[1]

During the first six months of 1966 only two coronary angiographies were carried out in London's important National Heart Hospital. This contrasts markedly with the figures previously mentioned from Cleveland, Ohio. In a recent report from the latter clinic the authors report that they had done 1,001 coronary angiographies between 1961 and 1964. This figure excludes those done on patients with valvular disease. A sur-

[1] G. Hale, D. Dexter, K. Jefferson and A. Leatham, of St. George's Hospital, London, *British Heart Journal*, 1966, **28**, 40.

prising statement is made in this review of the diagnostic accuracy of this investigation that the 1,000 coronary angiographies done prior to 1961 'are not considered because of technical or interpretative errors in the early experiments'.[1] At a symposium held at the Royal College of Physicians, London, in June 1966, Dr. Sones, of the Cleveland Clinic, stated that his unit had done 6,200 coronary angiographies with a mortality of six due to the procedure.[2]

My own personal opinion is that the submission of symptomless people to this complex and dramatic procedure, with its necessary team of doctors and complexity of instruments, is likely to produce in them an anxiety which their condition does not justify.

Indeed, what constitutes a minor and what a major complication is often a matter of personal opinion. The same applies to the consideration as to what constitutes a reasonable risk. As a former president of the Royal Society of Medicine remarked,[3]

> All experiments involve some risk. It may be an infinitesimally small one, but it is always there. If the experiment involves special techniques, then the risk is considerably enhanced.

In fact, to talk of completely innocuous experiments is a contradiction in terms. All experiments by their very nature must have unknown potentialities, otherwise they would not be experiments. The author of the last quotation has himself described how he volunteered to receive an apparently innocuous injection of pyrogen (a fever-producing substance). The effect on him was 'alarming', and he considers a subsequent attack of jaundice as being directly due to that experiment.

But when several different investigations, each with its own separate risk, are done simultaneously, then the possibilities of harm to the patient are proportionately, or more than proportionately, increased.

The usual method of obtaining blood samples is from a vein, but the reader will find many examples in this book referring to the insertion of needles or catheters into arteries. To the

[1] W. L. Proudfit, Earl Shirey and Mason Sones, Jr., of Cleveland Clinic, Ohio, *Circulation*, 1966, **33**, 901.
[2] Reported in *Medical Tribune of Great Britain*, June 1966.
[3] McCance, *Proceedings Royal Society Medicine*, 1951, **44**, 189.

experimenter this is often a very minor part of the whole procedure on which he is embarked. But even this part of the process is not free from the risk of unpleasant complications. Professor Mushin of the Welsh National School of Medicine recently pointed out in a letter to the *British Medical Journal*:

> That arterial puncture is so widely used leads to the assumption that it is a safe enough procedure for research purposes. There are, nevertheless, references in the literature to complications, although these are rarely specified, and there are still doubts in the minds of some whether this procedure is sufficiently free from serious complications to make its use justifiable for research purposes in patients for whom it is not strictly required for diagnosis or treatment. The patient's permission does not remove the need for this question to be clarified.[1]

Two doctors from a London teaching hospital who have had wide experience of arterial puncture have written:[2]

> This experience shows that arterial puncture commonly causes discomfort and may cause serious complications. It is 'safe' enough as a diagnostic procedure when the information it gives is essential for the patient's welfare, but it is not acceptable as a research procedure.

Yet, in spite of these influential opinions, a large proportion of the reports quoted in this book describe the insertion of a wide-bore needle, cannula or catheter into a femoral or brachial artery, as part, albeit a comparatively small part, of the experiment.

A doctor may have developed a certain technical skill, for example, in passing cardiac catheters or puncturing some viscus such as the liver or heart, so that after many performances he can now do so with hardly any risk of a patient dying and comparatively little risk of a major complication. While acquiring this skill there have almost certainly been major complications and even fatalities, but now that the technique has been more or less mastered, the chances of either are very much less. Does this justify him in continuing on many more patients for experimental purposes? I consider that the answer to this question is

[1] *British Medical Journal*, 1964, **2,** 310.
[2] Ikram and P. G. N. Nixon, of Charing Cross Hospital, London, *British Medical Journal*, 1964, **2,** 1072.

undoubtedly, 'No'. To cite one out of many possible examples, the technique of liver biopsy has been successfully developed in recent years, so that in expert hands this difficult and otherwise risky procedure can, generally speaking, be done safely. All the same, even those practised in this technique should only undertake to do it in circumstances which provide what is often called, in medical parlance, a 'real indication'. Professor Sherlock, a highly experienced leader in medical research experiments, has written:

> Needle biopsy of the liver should be regarded as potentially fatal. Five hundred biopsies may be performed without incident, only the five hundred and first to be complicated by massive intraperitoneal haemorrhage demanding immediate treatment. The patients must therefore be carefully selected and a real indication for it must be present before a biopsy is performed.[1]

What Professor Sherlock says here should apply to all investigations where risk to the patient is involved. But what constitutes a 'real indication'? Can an experiment the possible findings of which can be of no possible use in the treatment of the patient be said to be based on a 'real indication'? This is the core of the matter.

Mere technical virtuosity, often obtained at many patients' expense, can never justify its continued performance, simply because the operator has acquired that particular skill, simply because he may now be able to claim that the mortality rate in such experiments is only 0.1% and the risk of serious complications only 1%. And what of the other doctors who will later learn these techniques? They, too, will probably defend the procedure in question by claiming that the mortality rate is only 0.1%, though, in fact, it is likely to be much higher in their hands until they become experts.

Not only this. The figures of mortality and of the occurrence of major complications – what we may call the 'casualty figures' of medical experiments – are themselves, like the casualty figures in war, not always accurately reported. The figures quoted in medical literature only too frequently err on the side of understatement.

[1] *Journal of Clinical Pathology*, 1962, **15**, 291.

But a further important point has been stressed by a previously quoted authority,

> There have been instances in which certain details and complications have been deleted from published reports to avoid unfavourable criticism. It seems unlikely that such abuses are common, but when they occur it is probable that the study should not have been carried out in the first place. The failure to report serious complications in a final report is inexcusable.[1]

In 1942 Dr. Pendergrass of Philadelphia sent a questionnaire to a large number of radiologists asking about deaths which had occurred as a direct consequence of a comparatively innocuous method of visualizing the urinary tract known as intravenous pyelography.[2] In replies to his questionnaire, Dr. Pendergrass was notified of twenty-six deaths so caused, whereas only eleven had been reported in medical journals. In 1952 Dr. Terry of St. Bartholomew's Hospital, London, wrote that although up to that date only thirteen deaths from liver biopsy had been reported in medical journals, he personally knew of five other deaths due to the same procedure which had never been reported.[3] In 1953 the literature of liver puncture was reviewed and the thirty-nine fatal cases due to this procedure which had been reported up to that date, fully discussed. The writers of this review concluded that the frequency of complications and deaths is small, but added:

> There is abundant evidence that the frequency of serious complications, including death, is high in inexperienced hands. Unreported fatal cases are known to have occurred in the hands of inadequately trained personnel – it should not be undertaken casually . . . Less discriminate use of liver biopsy is accompanied by high morbidity and disastrous mortality.[4]

Indeed, Professor Sherlock in her own book on liver disease, has written that, 'Deaths due directly to diagnostic procedures are often not published.'[5]

[1] H. K. Beecher, Massachusetts General Hospital, Boston, Mass., *Journal American Medical Association*, 1959, **169,** 461.
[2] *American Journal of Roentgenology*, 1942, **48,** 741.
[3] *British Medical Journal*, 1952, **1,** 1102.
[4] Zamcheck and Klausenstock, of Boston, Mass., *New England Journal of Medicine* 1953, **249,** 1020, 1062.
[5] Sherlock, *Diseases of the Liver* (Blackwell), 1965.

The Risk to Patients

The procedure known as translumbar aortography necessitates turning the patient on to his face and stabbing a large needle to the side of the spinal column to a depth of six inches, so that it pierces the wall of the abdominal aorta (the main artery to the abdominal organs and also to the lower limbs). When the needle enters the lumen[1] of the aorta and blood spurts through the needle, a contrast medium is injected directly into the aorta so that it and its branches can be visualized on serial X-rays.

In an article published in 1957[2] an American radiologist noted that serious complications of this procedure had been reported, but added, 'The frequency of these unfortunate complications however is not known.' In an attempt to determine this he wrote to 450 radiologists in the U.S.A., but obtained complete replies from only 194. This private survey revealed thirty-seven deaths directly due to this investigation of which twelve were due to kidney damage, five to spinal-cord damage, and five to haemorrhage from the aorta. But in addition ninety-eight cases of serious but non-fatal complications were revealed, including twenty-four cases of resultant paralysis of both legs, twenty-seven cases of serious kidney damage and eight who suffered sequelae resulting from severe haemorrhage.

Three years later two other American radiologists[3] noted that up to that date there had been reported in the literature twenty-nine cases (five immediately fatal) of spinal cord damage with resultant paralysis of both legs as a direct consequence of this investigation. But a questionnaire sent to four hundred American radiologists revealed a further eighteen such cases, hitherto not published. So the figure for this terrible complication of translumbar aortography is at least forty-seven and not the twenty-nine usually quoted. The true incidence must, of course, be very much higher.

The same authors comment:

Instances of damage to almost every abdominal viscus, including kidney, pancreas, small bowel, gall bladder, colon, spleen,

---

[1] The *lumen* is the channel or space within a hollow tube such as a catheter and a blood-vessel or a tubular organ such as the colon.

[2] J. G. McAfee, of Johns Hopkins Hospital, Baltimore, *Radiology*, 1957, **68**, 825.

[3] Killen and J. H. Foster, of Vanderbilt School of Medicine, *Annals of Surgery*, 1960, **152**, 211.

adrenal, and ovary as well as to certain extra-abdominal organs, especially spinal cord and skin, have been encountered,

and give a large list of references substantiating this.

But the procedure has in addition another hazard which is much more difficult to assess, namely the effects of accidentally injecting the contrast medium into the wall of the aorta instead of its lumen. Any such deleterious effects may take a long time, even years, to become manifest. Such damage may result in weakening of the artery wall, which, as a consequence, becomes split or ballooned (dissection aneurysm). Commenting on this possibility, an English radiologist has written:[1]

> Subintimal injection of the contrast medium (i.e. into the arterial wall instead of the lumen) with resultant aortic dissection is a major hazard. . . . Even a small aortic dissection if strategically placed can have major consequences. . . . A major subintimal injection weakens the aortic wall which may rupture. It may tear off the origins of arteries, some of which may be vital end arteries, e.g. renal, mesenteric (to bowel), gonadal and spinal, with consequent necrosis of their supplied organs. Aortic dissection may also occlude the aortic lumen, resulting in impaired blood flow to the distal tissues.

Indeed, in a series of 425 consecutive translumbar aortographies performed in one American clinic[2] this complication, the accidental injection of the contrast medium into the aortic wall, occurred in forty-two (10%) of the patients. The authors comment:

> In three of these the death of the patient was directly or indirectly related to the intramural injection, two of the patients dying with proved dissecting aneurysms. The other 39 had no significant complications.

But in those thirty-nine, possible sequelae at a much later date cannot be ruled out.

Another fatality from translumbar aortography was recorded in 1962 in a patient where such a procedure was possibly justified. A thirty-one-year-old negress had abdominal pain and

[1] R. G. Grainger, of Sheffield, England, *British Journal of Radiology*, 1965, **38**, 201.
[2] Boblitt, M. M. Figley and E. F. Wolfman, University of Michigan Hospital, Ann Arbor, *Americab Journal Roentgenology*, 1959, **81**, 826.

urinary symptoms, and, because the diagnosis was in doubt, it was decided to submit her to aortography. However, the needle, instead of entering the abdominal aorta, was accidentally pushed into the spinal canal, and the contrast medium was injected into the meninges. Forty-five minutes later severe lumbar pain was followed by convulsions and the patient died in two hours. Post-mortem showed a tuberculous left kidney, which could have been successfully treated.[1]

Obviously, many experimenters are willing to take risks. But, although when discussing this some seem to regard the risk chiefly as a danger to their personal reputations, or of the possibility of legal action against themselves, the real risk is, of course, the patient's. Professor McCance has said:

> I do not think I would have had the temerity to carry out the first hepatic or cardiac catheterization. The risk in any experiment depends very much on whether the investigator knows that he will always retain control of the situation. To inoculate somebody with ictogenic serum (an injection of blood which will produce jaundice) is a risk that I personally would never take, nor would I ever have cared to take it even before the risks were so well known, for once the inoculation had taken place I would have lost control.[2]

Many investigators who inject foreign substances into people forget the important fact that, once having given the injection, they may be unable to control its effects, as Professor McCance so rightly points out.

A non-medical has put the case even stronger:

> There is the obvious fact that some human being will always be the first one upon whom a medical technique is tested or to whom a new medicine will be administered. But the question is, 'When is it morally justified to use the first human being for experimental purposes?'[3]

I would like to emphasize that in this book, with but very few exceptions, only experiments which have been recorded in medical journals are discussed. Undoubtedly, and for obvious

[1] Doroshov, Young Yoon, M. A. Robbins, of Sinai Hospital, Baltimore, *Journal Urology*, 1962, **88**, 439.

[2] *Proceedings of the Royal Society of Medicine*, 1951, **44**, 189.

[3] S. E. Stumpf, Department of Philosophy, Vanderbilt University, Nashville, Tennessee, *Annals of Internal Medicine*, 1966, **64**, 460.

reasons, the worst experiments go unrecorded. That this is so is borne out by information given me by numerous postgraduate students of mine who have told me of what they themselves have witnessed. One such case concerns a London hospital where an experimental physician wished to practise the technique of lumbar aortography (described previously). The subjects chosen for this experiment were eight patients who had been admitted with gastric ulcers, most of them complicated by haemorrhage from the ulcer. The procedure was carried out in the X-ray department and the patients were obviously under the impression that it was part of the business of taking X-rays of their stomachs. As a direct result of the experimental procedure three out of these eight patients died.

There is one further point regarding risk and the rights of the patient and those of the doctor. Though not everyone will agree, the view should be heard that even a willing and informed patient may not be morally justified in accepting certain risks. It can be maintained that everyone has a certain moral obligation *not* to run undue risks with his own health or life. The late Pope Pius XII expressed this view when, in addressing an international medical congress in September 1952, he said that,

> . . . The patient, then, has no right to involve his physical or psychic integrity in medical experiments or research when they entail serious destruction, mutilation, wounds or perils.

In the great majority of articles giving accounts of experiments on people, including most of those reported in this book, the authors do not mention whether consent was obtained. Therefore, in any particular example cited, unless definitely stated to the contrary, we must not assume that valid consent was, or was not, given. We do not know the truth.

It must be appreciated that it may be difficult to draw a sharp distinction between an investigation done in the patient's own interest, for the diagnosis or assessment of his own condition, and a purely experimental research investigation. This is especially true when the patient is suffering from the disease process being investigated. A great deal of the research into heart, liver and kidney disease is of this nature. The value to any individual patient of some of this type of investigation is often problematical, and this is especially so if the procedure is in any way novel. Some research doctors take advantage of this ambiguity, and this is likely to be particularly true in those hospitals where a multiplication of investigations is regarded as 'routine'.

4. THE PRINCIPLE OF MEDICAL MORALITY

Many experiments are defended by those who carry them out on the grounds that, while admittedly of no help to the patient or other person who is the subject, the aim of such experiments is ultimately to help mankind. My contention is that it is immoral to perform experiments, especially dangerous ones, on unsuspecting patients not suffering from the disease being investigated, solely in the hope of making scientific discoveries. Science is not the ultimate good, and the pursuit of new scientific knowledge should not be allowed to take precedence over moral values where the two are in conflict. The statement which is not uncommonly heard among research workers, 'It would be interesting to know', though natural and, doubtless, frequently true, is not in itself a justification for making experiments of whatever kind. The welfare of the subject must also and always be taken into account.

Any human being has the right to be treated with a certain decency, and this right, which is individual, supersedes every consideration of what may benefit science or contribute to the public welfare. No physician is justified in placing science or the public welfare first and his obligation to the individual, who is his patient or subject, second. No doctor, however great his capacity or original his ideas, has the right to choose martyrs for science or for the general good. Over a hundred years ago a famous French doctor who is regarded by many as the real founder of modern experimental medicine, Claude Bernard, put it thus:

> The principle of medical morality consists then in never performing on man an experiment which could be harmful to him in any degree whatsoever though the result may be of great interest to science, that is, of benefit to save the health of others.[1]

[1] *Introduction à l'Étude de la Médecine Expérimentale*, 1856. (A new translation of this book by H. C. Greene was published in 1962 by Abelard-Schuman.)

Introduction

That this principle has been greatly transgressed, as a recent editorial in the *British Medical Journal* has pointed out,[1] does not confute its truth. Indeed, the fact that very great advances, and recent ones, have been made in medical research which has in no way offended against this principle, is all the more grounds for observing it. The introduction of the insulin treatment of diabetes[2] and of liver treatment of pernicious anaemia[3] (both of which diseases were previously fatal) were arrived at through research which did not come to its findings by means of distressing, risky and sometimes fatal experiments on human subjects. Nor were there any extensive controlled clinical trials prior to the successful establishment of penicillin.

An American philosopher has put the position clearly:

> One cannot therefore justify any and every act in the name of the common good and therefore not every use of human beings in research can be justified in the broad notion that in the end others will benefit from such experiments. We must approach the concept of the greater good with our other three affirmations always in mind; that we must protect life, that health is better than sickness, and that we treat individuals as persons and not simply as means.[4]

An American physician has stated the matter even more strongly:[5]

> Any classification of human experimentation as 'for the good of society' is to be viewed with distaste, even alarm. Undoubtedly, all sound work has this as its ultimate aim, but such high-flown expressions are not necessary, and have been used within living memory as cover for outrageous ends.

[1] *British Medical Journal*, 1962, 2, 1108. The editorial, in speaking of the above treatise by Claude Bernard said, 'It should be read at least by those whose enthusiasm for investigation seems at times to run into conflict with the obligations as physicians in charge of patients', and added that since the time Bernard wrote, 'Hundreds and hundreds of experiments have been conducted which conflict with the principles of medical morality or medical ethics, as enunciated by the founder of experimental medicine.'

[2] By Banting and Best in 1921.

[3] By Minot and Murphy in 1926.

[4] S. E. Stumpf, of Department of Philosophy, Vanderbilt University, Nashville, Tennessee, *Annals of Internal Medicine*, 1966, 64, 460.

[5] H. K. Beecher in *Clinical Investigation – Medical, Ethical, and Moral Aspects* (Boston University Press, 1963).

Part I

WHAT IS BEING DONE

Almost every category of human subject submitted to a medical experiment has a peculiar call on the considerateness of the doctors in charge of that experiment and of anyone else who shares responsibility for it. Every patient who becomes an experimental subject, for instance, is entitled to special consideration simply by virtue of the fact that, being a patient, he or she is a sick person. The same applies, I think, to a woman who is pregnant, to a mental defective or someone who is mentally ill, to a man in prison, to an old person, and to anyone whose disease is fatal, progressive and incurable (in other words, who is dying). It also applies to a volunteer who is in good health, but who, as such volunteers often are, is in a dependent relationship to the doctors conducting the experiment; and I would say, even, that it applies when the experimenter uses himself as his subject.

But when experimenting on somebody else, then the research worker has the responsibility for the welfare of the subject used. The exact nature of this responsibility will vary with the category of patient. Therefore I will discuss separately experiments on different categories of patients and try to indicate what are the special considerations due to each group. Obviously these groups are not mutually exclusive and there is much overlap.

The special considerations that should be given to children and infants are, first, that they are particularly vulnerable and helpless and therefore call for more consideration than other groups. Secondly, a child cannot give consent to any experiment. In medical circles it is often considered an adequate safeguard if both parents have given consent after full explanation and avowal of methods and possible consequences. But in actual fact the law both here and in America appears to be very definite, namely, that parents, either singly or together, cannot give valid legal consent to any action that is not for the immediate benefit of the child concerned. A leading American lawyer has stated quite unequivocally:

31

Parents cannot consent unless the invasion of the child's body is for the child's welfare or benefit.[1]

In law, minors rank as children.

Let us begin with two experiments in which those responsible were criticized, and, in reply, defended their procedures. The two reports were in the same issue of a medical journal. The first experiment[2] was to investigate the safety of giving ammonium chloride intravenously in large amounts to children. As subjects for the experiment two four-month-old hydrocephalic ('water on the brain') infants were used and this procedure was tried out first on them.

The purpose of the second experiment[3] was to explore the relationship between a rare disease, phenylketonuria, which causes retardation of physical and mental development, and the presence of phenylketone derivatives in the diet. The child subjected to this experiment was aged two and is described as, 'an idiot, unable to stand, walk or talk'.

The child was given a special diet free of all phenylketone derivatives, and after ten months' treatment showed a marked improvement. After discharge from hospital, but keeping on the special diet, she continued to improve. But, in order to rule out the possibility that the improvement was spontaneous, the infant was readmitted to hospital and 'without the mother's knowledge' she was put on a diet with large amounts of phenylketone. The report notes,

> The mother reported with distress that her daughter had lost in a few days all the good gained in the previous 10 months.

Incidentally, the authors mention that prior to giving the infant the pheynylketone they first tried its effects on a normal five-month-old baby to prove that it was safe.

These two reports evoked a protest which was published in the next issue of the journal.

A correspondent wrote apropos of both experiments:[4]

[1] Professor F. A. Freund, of Harvard Law School, *New England Journal of Medicine*, 1965, **273**, 687.
[2] Doxiadis, Goldfinch and Holt, of Children's Hospital, Sheffield, *Lancet*, 1953, **2**, 801.
[3] Bickel, Garrard and Hickmans, of Children's Hospital, Birmingham, England, *Lancet*, 1953, **2**, 812.
[4] R. E. W. Fisher, *Lancet*, 1953, **2**, 993.

Experiments on Infants and Children

It is a matter for regret that the use of normal children, or children suffering from some irrelevent disease, as controls in clinical research appears to be increasing. No medical procedure involving the slightest risk or accompanied by the slightest physical or mental pain may be inflicted on a child for experimental purposes unless there is a reasonable chance, or at least a hope, that that child may benefit thereby.

The defence of the first group of experimenters was,[1]

Our own working policy is that no procedure should be carried out involving risk or discomfort without a reasonable chance of benefit to that child *or other children* [their italics].

In rebuttal of this defence another doctor replied,[2]

There is no justification here for risking an injury to an individual for the possible benefit to other people, as enunciated by them as their guiding principle. Such a rule would open the door wide to perversions of practice, even such as were inflicted by the Nazi doctors on concentration camp prisoners.

The defence of the second group of experimenters was: 'The phenylketone test was comparable to a glucose tolerance test done on a diabetic.' But this comparison is valid only if it is stipulated that the glucose tolerance test is done on a known severe diabetic. But no clinician who respected his patient would do such a test, because of its possibly serious consequences. I consider that the analogy thus breaks down and with it their defence.

In 1954 heart catheterization was performed on sixteen children, aged eleven to sixteen, and one adult aged twenty,[3] ten of whom had active rheumatic heart disease, while the other seven were recovering from acute rheumatic fever. In the latter group the disease was considered to be inactive, although four had valvular disease.

The experiment consisted in passing a catheter, under X-ray control, via the main arm vein into the subclavian vein of the chest, thence into the superior vena cava, thence into the right

[1] Ibid.
[2] D. Leys, *Lancet*, 1953, **2**, 1044.
[3] Besterman at Taplow Hospital, Bucks., England, *British Heart Journal*, 1954, **16**, 8.

atrium of the heart, and so into the pulmonary artery (see diagram). At the same time a tightly fitting face mask and nose clip were applied to each child's face, so that samples of air breathed out could be collected for analysis. After blood samples had been taken from the heart (through the catheter) and pressure recordings within the heart were obtained, the children were made to 'cycle' on a special machine, and they did this with the cardiac catheter and face mask remaining in position.

The conclusion reached as a result of this experiment was: 'Active rheumatic carditis interferes with the functional efficiency of the heart.' This fact, however, was not only already well known but was well established. The purpose of the experiment had been, as is so often the case in experimental medicine, merely to confirm some existing knowledge.

The same physician described another experiment[1] which was done with a colleague, in which cardiac catheterization was carried out on fifteen children suffering from acute rheumatic fever complicated by pericardial effusion (fluid accumulating between the two membrances covering the heart). This is a very serious condition, which can be gauged from the fact that the author himself had recorded a mortality of 50% in thirty of his own cases.[2]

The report states:

Two of them with large effusions were catheterized in order to confirm the value of the technique.

In fact, in only six of the children was the diagnosis in doubt, and this means that nine very sick children were subjected to this unpleasant, risky and possibly frightening procedure in order to confirm the validity of a means of diagnosis which in their case was superfluous.

In the two experiments just described the children were suffering from a disease affecting the heart. But in two other experiments described below heart catheterizations were carried out on very young infants who were, in the words of the report, 'free from cardiac defect'.[3] The aim of these experiments

[1] Besterman and G. T. Thomas, at Taplow Hospital, Bucks., England, *British Heart Journal*, 1953, **15**, 113.
[2] Besterman, *British Heart Journal*, 1953, **15**, 29.
[3] R. D. Rowe and L. S. James, of Toronto Hospital for Sick Children and Columbia Presbyterian Medical Centre, N.Y., *Journal of Paediatrics*, 1957, **51**, 1.

was to determine normal pressures in the pulmonary artery during the first few months of life.

The first experiment was carried out on fifteen mentally defective infants aged between two days and nine months. The catheter was passed via the saphenous vein of the thigh, through the main veins of the abdomen and chest, through the heart and thence into the pulmonary artery. At the same time a cannula (a very large hollow needle) was inserted into, and kept in, the femoral artery of the other thigh. It is recorded that no sedative was given prior to the experiment.

The second experiment was done by the same physicians on thirteen mentally deficient infants, all of them less than twelve months old, none of whom had any recognizable signs of heart disease and some of whom had been included in the previous study. With these thirteen, catheters were passed to the heart by the same route. In this experiment, however, the infants were fitted with tight face masks and made to breathe a gas mixture which was 90% nitrogen. Nitrogen is an irrespirable gas, and the purpose of this part of the experiment was to produce a condition called hypoxia – a gross interference with respiration resulting from insufficient oxygen in the blood. While hypoxia was sustained by this means, blood samples were taken from the heart (through the catheter), and were again taken when the 90% nitrogen mixture had been replaced by making the infants inhale 100% oxygen. It is recorded:

> When the saturation of oxygen fell to below 40% the infants began to move and become restless, finally crying strenuously, sometimes in a gasping fashion. One infant had a period of apnoea (cessation of breathing).

A few years later an experimental study by means of cardiac catheterization was made on an even younger group of subjects. The physicians seem to have been motivated by the fact that to their knowledge no such studies had so far been made on a large scale, and undertook the following experiment with thirty-eight newborn infants, none of whom had heart disease.[1] The experiment was done on these infants within thirty hours of birth. Of

[1] A. M. Rudolph, Drorbough, P. A. M. Auld, A. J. Rudolph, Nadas, C. A. Smith and Hubbell, of Lying-in Hospital and Children's Medical Center, Boston, Mass., *Pediatrics*, 1961, **27,** 551.

the thirty-eight subjects nineteen, among whom were five mental defectives, were free from respiratory disease; nine had mild respiratory distress; ten had 'severe respiratory distress'. The severity of this condition may be judged from the fact that eight of these ten died between three and fifty-eight hours of the completition of the experiment, their deaths being caused by a lung condition known as 'Hyaline Membrane Disease', and not primarily as a direct result of the procedure.

The experiment was as follows. A catheter was passed either through the saphenous vein of the leg or through the umbilical vein and thence through the main veins of the abdomen and chest into the heart. In twenty cases the catheter was passed beyond the right side of the heart into the left side. With at least fifteen of the infants two attempts to perform the catheterization were necessary. No anaesthetics or any pre-medication were used. However, the nineteen, who were suffering from respiratory disease before the experiment had begun, were given oxygen throughout the procedure. The authors' comment on the question of consent by the parents of these babies was:

> The decision to perform the studies on the infants was made after careful clinical observation. The procedure was performed after full discussion and consent of at least one of the parents.

An investigation by a catheterization technique into the heart output of newborn babies was carried out in 1955. This was done on twenty-nine healthy infants aged from two to twenty-six hours.[1]

A recent repetition of this investigation was carried out in Australia, but using more complex and sophisticated techniques. The experiment was done on twenty-seven healthy newborn infants aged from two to twenty-eight hours. A special feeding tube (technically described as a number five, French) was passed via an umbilical artery at the navel into the descending aorta. Pressures were recorded and blood samples taken. This tube was then withdrawn. A special electrical instrument for measuring blood temperature, called a thermistor, was mounted at the tip of a length of tiflon, and this was threaded through a

[1] Klara Prec and D. E. Cassels, of University Chicago Clinics, *Circulation*, 1955, **11**, 789.

rubber seal and lucite adapter and then drawn on to a poly-thene catheter. This thermistor and catheter assembly were then passed through the umbilical artery into the aorta. Another feeding-tube was then passed via the umbilical vein and great veins into the left atrial heart chamber. Blood samples were taken from the aorta and the heart and three injections of saline were given through the heart catheter (five in some infants) and further samples were taken. The catheter was then withdrawn from the heart. Another catheter was then passed into the other umbilical artery until it rested in the aorta eight to ten centi-metres above the thermistor. The experiment was then com-pleted by fitting a clip and valve mechanism to the infant's nose so as to collect samples of expired air during the following three to four minutes. The consent of the parents is neither mentioned nor discussed.[1]

A more difficult and more hazardous method of cardiac investigation is done by means of what is known as retrograde left-sided catheterization. Here, instead of being passed along a vein in the same direction as the blood flow, the catheter is passed along the artery *against* the blood flow, and by this route into the left ventricle of the heart. This procedure was carried out on the children whose ages ranged from three months to nineteen years. Five of them were suffering from valvular lesions; the other five were free from heart disease.[2]

The procedure consisted in passing a catheter 'of the widest possible diameter' through the main artery of the left arm after making an incision over the artery and in the artery wall. Thence the catheter was passed (against the blood stream) into the subclavian artery in the chest, thence into the aorta and through the aortic valve into the left ventricle of the heart. The whole procedure was done under X-ray control, a contrast medium being injected through the catheter so that the heart and the great vessels would show in clear outline on the X-ray films. When the experiment was finished the artery wall that had been initially incised had to be sutured (stitched).

The authors of the report, commenting on the use of the five

---

[1] E. D. Burnard, A. Grauaug and R. E. Gray, of Women's Hospital, Sydney, *Clinical Science*, 1966, **31**, 121.

[2] Arcilla, Agustsson, Steiger and Gasul, of Cook County Hospital, Chicago, Illinois, *Circulation*, 1961, **23**, 269.

children who were free from heart disease, say that in their case the experiment 'was performed to investigate some other extra-cardiac disorder'. No details of such disorders are, however, given, and I am unaware of any conditions which would justify what was done. Retrograde cardiac catheterization is a procedure which requires great skill and invariably involves grave hazards. The authors' comment, 'The method is not devoid of difficulties', seriously understates the hazards.

In order to establish the normal values for cerebral blood flow in children the following experiment on nine children aged three to eleven was carried out.[1] No other details about the children are given except the fact that they did not have brain disease. Twelve adults, about whom no details are recorded, were used as controls.

First, a needle was inserted into the femoral artery (the main artery of the thigh). Second, the jugular vein (the main vein of the neck) was punctured deeply by another needle just below the angle of the jaw so that this needle could penetrate to the bulb of this vein. Third, while these two needles were in position the patient was made to inhale a special gas mixture through a tightly fitting face mask.

I quote the above case because, apart from the unpleasantness of the procedure, the experimenters themselves underline what they were doing when they make four observations. The first is the note that 'to minimize the pain in obtaining blood samples very sharp needles were used'. The second is that two three-year-olds who were among those submitted to the experiment 'required some restraint'. The third is that the children's legs were immobilized by bandaging them to a board. The fourth is that '*thirty-five others* were originally selected for the procedure, but at one stage or another they became unco-operative'.

Vincent's angina is a severe infection of the mouth which produces ulceration of the gums, tonsils and inside the cheeks. Some physicians attempted to transmit this disease from infected children to others with healthy mouths. The mouths of the infected children were swabbed and the material was put on to the gums and tonsils of eleven children with healthy

[1] C. Kennedy and Sokoloff, of Children's Hospital, Philadelphia, *Journal Clinical Investigation*, 1957, **36**, 1131.

mouths. In view of the negative results obtained, a further fourteen children with healthy mouths had their gums and tonsils mechanically traumatized by rubbing prior to the application of the infected material to these areas.[1]

In 1949 it was decided to investigate the possibility of toxic effects from agene, a substance which is used as an 'improver' in the manufacture of flour.[2] There had been many reports of its toxic effects in animals and the purpose of the study was to see if similar effects were liable to occur in human beings. As the authors state,

> The knowledge that in dogs excessive doses cause ataxia (clumsiness of movement), disorientation, epilepsy, and haemorrhagic lesions of the bowel, gave little indication of the effects that were to be expected in man.
> With the co-operation of the local authority concerned, such an investigation was undertaken on eighty boys, aged ten to fifteen, in a residential school. Almost all the children came from homes which were social failures; they were, however, free from gross physical or mental defects.

The boys were split into two groups. One was put on a diet with agene-free flour and the other on a diet with agenized flour. These diets were continued for six months, and the two groups were then switched. When it was found that the agene did not have any toxic effects, two adult volunteers were put on a diet containing larger amounts of agene for six weeks.

In 1953 an experiment was carried out which involved the deliberate blistering of the abdomen of forty-one children, aged eight- to fourteen, by the application of an irritant, cantharides.[3] The purpose was to assess the variable severity of the response, and this was done by removing the fluid from the blisters, which were about one square inch, and to measure its volume accurately. Thirty of the children had rheumatic fever and in them the blistering was done before and after treatment. These results were compared with those from a group of five children

[1] J. Schartzman and Leo Grossman, of Metropolitan Hospital, New York City, *Archives Pediatrics*, 1941, **58**, 515.
[2] A. Elithorn, Doris Johnson (non-medical) and Margaret Crosskey (non-medical), from National Hospital, Nervous Diseases, London, *Lancet*, 1949, **1**, 143.
[3] Barbara Ansell, Antinini and L. E. Glynn, of Taplow Hospital, Bucks., England, *Clinical Science*, 1953, **12**, 367.

ill with other diseases, and another group of six described as 'healthy normal controls'. This last group were subjected to blistering on three separate occasions.

The author's own description of the technique is interesting.

> Blister skin was removed with scissors, the raw area swabbed with peroxide and covered with oiled silk. Healing occurred in 5 to 6 days, leaving a small pigmented area.

One of the first reported tests of the safety of live poliomyelitis virus for use in immunization came from America in 1952. The live virus was given to twenty patients who are described as volunteers, but an enigmatic footnote states,

> For obvious reasons the age, sex and physical status of these volunteers are not mentioned.

In fact, none of the patients developed paralytic poliomyelitis.[1]

In 1963 the following experiment on 113 newborn infants, aged one to seventy-seven hours, of whom twenty-six had been premature births, was undertaken.[2] In thirteen the experiment was unsuccessful. The authors wrote, 'In each case the procedure was discussed in detail with one or both parents, followed by written consent'. They state, 'All the infants were in good condition', and that when, without prior premedication, a catheter was passed via the umbilical artery into the infant's aorta, 'with few exceptions the infants appeared to be completely content'.

We are told, however, 'pressures were recorded in the descending aorta both at rest and during crying', the second period being presumably at a time when these infants were not quite so 'completely content'. After catheterization of the thoracic aorta, the procedure varied. On forty-six of the infants, of whom seventeen had been premature, 'cold pressor' tests were done.

The procedure was to immerse one of the infant's feet in iced water for one minute, and the aortic pressure was recorded during the immersion and thereafter for two to five minutes. The report states, 'Since the infants invariably cried when ex-

---

[1] Koprowski, G. A. Jervis and T. W. Norton, of Lederle Research Laboratory, Pearl River, New York, *American Journal Hygiene*, 1952, **55,** 108.

[2] Moss, Duffie and Emmanouilides, of Department of Pediatrics, University of California, *Pediatrics*, 1963, **32,** 175.

posed to cold, one to three pretest immersions at one minute intervals were made until all signs of discomfort disappeared'.

The effects of tilting on aortic pressure were studied in a further fifty infants, of whom twenty-three were premature.

The subjects were secured to a board with the upper extremities restrained in flexion and the lower in extension. The board was then tilted over the edge of a table. Tilting did not usually cause any signs of discomfort. When it did, the test was repeated until a satisfactory pressure recording was obtained.

A new method of X-ray visualization of the infant's heart was described in 1963.[1] The subjects were ten infants aged one to ten days, all of whom were 'in poor to critical condition', because of severe congenital heart lesions, and nine of them were cyanozed (blue). Catheters were passed via the umbilical vein into the vena cava and so into the heart. In the older infants an incision had to be made over the navel to isolate the umbilical vein. In four cases the catheter was passed via the umbilical artery instead of the vein and thus into the aorta before it entered the heart. In all the infants a contrast medium was injected via the catheter and serial X-rays taken. Three deaths occurred within twenty-four hours of this procedure, but these, says the report, 'were felt to be due to the underlying disease rather than the study itself.'

An experiment in India has been described in which a considerable percentage of the subjects were children.[2] The purpose of the experiment was to confirm (which was already known) that patients with a congenital anomaly of their red blood cells known as Thalassaemia, which gives rise to a special type of severe anaemia, have an increased resistance to malaria. Eighteen patients with Thalassaemia were the subjects and also a control group of fourteen patients who had anaemia due to different causes.

Both groups were injected with blood from other patients who were ill with malaria. One result of the experiment was that the patients' anaemia became worse. The question of consent is not mentioned in the report.

[1] Sapin, Linde and Emmanouilides, of Department of Pediatrics, University of California, *Pediatrics*, 1963, **31**, 946.
[2] R. N. Ray, J. B. Chatterjea and R. N. Chaudhuri, of the School of Tropical Medicine, Calcutta, India, in *Bulletin of the World Health Organisation*, 1964, **30**, 51.

What is Being Done

The following descriptions illustrate the problem of forming a judgment as to the ethical correctness or otherwise of some experiments. The same difficulty applies to many of the experiments illustrated in this book. A severe form of a chronic insidious kidney disease, known as chronic pyelonephritis, has rightly received a good deal of attention during the last few years; its marked frequency has been noted, and its possible causations discussed.

One of its possible causes is a condition known as vesico (bladder)-ureteric reflux. The ureters are the two hollow tubes which convey urine from the kidneys to the bladder and each pierces the musculature of the bladder wall in an oblique direction, thus acting as a valve preventing urine from the bladder being forced back into the ureter when the full bladder contracts to void its urine. Should this mechanism be defective the resultant condition is known as vesico-ureteric reflux.

It was considered important to establish whether or not such reflux occurred in normal people, including infants. For this purpose a catheter was passed into the bladder, a dye was injected into it and then serial X-rays were taken, including some before, after and during micturition. This was performed on five normal people ranging in age from three to eighteen.[1] The same author, a year later, repeated the experiment on twenty-four normal people with an age range from nine months to seventy-four years, sixteen of whom were under eighteen. All the adults were submitted to cystoscopy, examination of the bladder with an illuminating telescopic instrument, prior to the investigation. A note states, 'If too young to co-operate, the catheter was indwelling and clamped'. No medical details of these 'normal' people are given.[2]

The author then proceeded to repeat the experiment on twenty-four pregnant women, of whom one was only sixteen and another seventeen. The exposure of these women to radiation of their pelvis cannot be discounted as of no importance, a point which will be discussed in more detail in a later section.

These reports appeared to show that without doubt vesico-ureteric reflux does not occur in normal people. Not content with this demonstration, two other doctors four years later re-

[1] R. G. Bunge, of Iowa College of Medicine, *Journal of Urology*, 1953, **70**, 729.
[2] R. G. Bunge, of Iowa College of Medicine, *Journal of Urology*, 1954, **71**, 427.

peated the investigation on 100 children with an age range of fourteen days to fourteen years, with an average of three and a half years. The only details otherwise given concerning these children is that they had no evidence of bladder or kidney disease and that the investigation was, 'Done following recovery from their illness when they were ready for discharge.'[1]

Only one of these children showed 'reflux'. A more recent review of the literature of this subject shows that there are published reports of this procedure having been done for purely experimental purposes on 330 children under the age of fourteen years who themselves had no suspicion of bladder or kidney disease.[2]

All reports, and the reader should again note their repetitious nature, go to prove that vesico-ureteric reflux does not occur in normal people. There is no doubt that this is an important point. It could be argued that it was essential to establish this, including in infants and pregnant women. But, even if this is agreed, there must be questioning concerning the ethics of the way in which this was established. Would the experimenter submit his infant or pregnant wife to this procedure so that possible light may be thrown on the cause of chronic pyelonephritis in others and so that sufferers from that disease may possibly be helped?

It must be clear from these accounts that the special consideration due to children and babies because of their particular vulnerability and helplessness is sometimes not given. And it must also be clear that the doctor's obligation to the parents and guardians regarding the asking of consent is not always carried out. In cases where an indefensible experiment is conducted *without* such consent a wrong has been done to both parent and child.

2. EXPERIMENTS ON PREGNANT WOMEN

The doctor's obligation towards a pregnant woman, like that towards a young child, is again a double one. It is to the expectant mother *and* to the unborn child. While a risk to the mother does not necessarily mean a risk to the child she will deliver, it

[1] B. W. Jones and J. W. Headstream, of University of Alabama, Medical Center, Little Rock, Arkansas, *Journal of Urology*, 1958, **80**, 114.

[2] *Journal of Urology*, 1960, **83**, 122.

should be remembered that a risk involving the child (or the foetus as it then is) may involve the mother's happiness even if, in a procedure which by some accident or bad luck injures the child, the mother herself is unharmed. The pregnant woman is *always* involved in any risk attached to an experiment of which she is made the subject; while the child is sometimes involved.

In 1949, when that procedure was still novel, cardiac catheterization was carried out on a hundred and six women subjects, the procedure being unsuccessful in ten cases.[1] Of the ninety-six successful cases, eighty-four were pregnant, four had been recently delivered, and eight, who were used as controls, were neither pregnant nor recently delivered. None of the subjects suffered from heart disease.

The authors of the report state that, 'All previous authors agree that cardiac output is increased in pregnancy.' The purpose of the investigation was to establish at which stage of pregnancy this happens. Ninety of the subjects were admitted from the antenatal clinic solely for the purpose of the investigation. They came into the hospital in the evening, underwent cardiac catheterization (without X-ray control) the following morning, and were discharged the same afternoon. Six of the subjects were already in the hospital for obstetric reasons. The authors of the report state, 'The procedure was explained to each patient and all volunteered.'

In the same journal a similar investigation is reported which was carried out in another hospital.[2] The subjects were seventy-five pregnant women, free from heart disease, the pregnancies ranging from six to forty weeks, and, in addition, thirty-two non-pregnant women who were used as controls. Of the pregnant it is stated, 'The majority volunteered from the antenatal clinic'.

In contrast to the previous experiment, the cardiac catheterization to which these subjects were submitted was done under X-ray control. The hazard of exposing pregnant women to radiation, especially in the early months, is not mentioned. The report does mention, however, that three of the subjects

[1] Alice Palmer and A. H. C. Walker, of Hammersmith Hospital, London, *Journal of Obstetrics and Gynaecology* (Britain), 1949, **56,** 537.
[2] Hiliary Hamilton, of Maternity Unit, Royal Infirmary, Edinburgh, *Journal of Obstetrics and Gynaecology*, 1949, **56,** 548.

were 'obviously apprehensive'. It is also recorded that one patient, after being catheterized, was found to have a haemoglobin[1] of only 50% of normal. In her case the results were therefore discarded. But it is very surprising that this patient's marked anaemia was not noticed before she was submitted to cardiac catheterization. One is also surprised that the experimenter, who had, in fact, learned the technique at the hospital in which the previous experiment was done, appears to have been unaware that a similar investigation was being carried out in her former hospital. Such unnecessary duplication of research studies is, unfortunately, a very common happening in experimental medicine.

The following investigation, of which the purpose was to study the effect of different postures on the cardiac output in the case of pregnant women, was done in 1961.[2] Thirty-one women who were in the last stages of pregnancy, described as Caucasians and negresses, were chosen. Five non-pregnant women, about whom no further details are given, were used as controls. The procedure was as follows. A needle was inserted into the brachial artery of one arm, and a catheter into the large vein of the other. This catheter was then passed into the thorax as far as the superior vena cava. Through the catheter a dye was injected. Four measurements of cardiac output were made with each patient in each of four postures. The postures were:

(1) horizontal;
(2) the patient lying on her side;
(3) the patient on her back with head and chest tilted backwards and downwards to an angle of 45°;
(4) the patient on her back with legs hanging over the side of the table.

An experiment was carried out on thirty-six normal women who were from fourteen to forty weeks pregnant, and another group of eleven who were from thirty-six to forty weeks pregnant. One was only fifteen; three only eighteen and two nineteen years of age.[3]

---

[1] Haemoglobin is the colouring matter of the red blood corpuscles of the blood.

[2] Vorys, Ullery and Hanusek, of Obstetrical Unit, Ohio State University, *American Journal of Obstetrics and Gynaecology*, 1961, **82**, 1312.

[3] R. A. Bader, M. E. Bader, D. J. Rose and E. Braunwald, of Mount Sinai Hospital, New York, *Journal Clinical Investigation*, 1955, **34**, 1524.

What is Being Done

All were subjected to cardiac catheterization under X-ray control, the catheter being passed through the heart into a small branch of the pulmonary artery. A large needle was inserted into the brachial artery, and, in addition the patients were fitted with tight face masks so that respiratory function could be measured simultaneously with heart function. When these had been completed, however, and with the cardiac catheter in position, the patients were made to work the pedals of a special bicycle for ten minutes.

The report states,

> No studies were performed prior to the 14th week of gestation because of the possible deleterious effect of radiation (X-rays) on the foetus.

This should be an essential safeguard, but is one which is frequently disregarded by experimentalists.

In order to determine the blood flow in the liver during pregnancy, a group of doctors passed cardiac catheters through the heart into the inferior vena cava and so into the hepatic vein of the liver of fifteen pregnant women in various stages of pregnancy, including two at full term. The experiment was repeated on six women with toxaemias of pregnancy, and a control series of fifteen non-pregnant women who were in the gynaecological ward.[1]

A group of physicians[2] decided to investigate the blood flow to the kidneys of pregnant women. Five normal pregnant women, all in the later stages of pregnancy were used. At 4 p.m. the women were given a meal of peanut butter, biscuits and raisins, but were not allowed any fluid. No food or drink was then permitted until the experiment was completed late the following morning. The first procedure was to pass a catheter into the bladder and this was kept there for the whole of the experiment. Intravenous infusions of two test substances were then given and blood and urine samples collected at frequent intervals. The patients were then given a high spinal anaesthetic. This involves sticking a needle into the spine and injecting

---

[1] Equina Munnell and Howard Taylor, of Bellevue Hospital, New York, *Journal Clinical Investigation*, 1947, **26,** 952.

[2] Assali, Kaplan, Foman, Douglass and Tada, of Cincinnati General Hospital, *Journal Clinical Investigation*, 1951, **30,** 916.

through this an anaesthetic, so as to induce loss of sensation and paralysis of the lower limbs, both of which will spread to the abdomen and chest if the patient is tilted. The patient is awake throughout this.

Spinal anaesthesia is not a pleasant procedure for any patient and has well-recognized dangers. These become more likely the higher the paralysis is made to spread by the tilting. In three of these five subjects, it is recorded that the effects of the spinal anaesthetic reached the fourth cervical segment of the spinal cord, which is very high and is likely to result in paralysis of the diaphragm.

After the spinal anaesthesia had been induced, the renal function tests were repeated. This revealed that the spinal anaesthesia had produced a considerable lowering of renal efficiency, an effect which could not possibly have been to the patients' advantage.

Justification for submitting these patients to the spinal anaesthetics is given in the following terms:

> High spinal blockade in the normal pregnant women affords
> a unique opportunity of studying the response of renal function
> to a marked drop in blood pressure, since this drop is not
> obtained in the normal non-pregnant individual.

A group of Cuban doctors not only gave spinal anaesthetics to a group of pregnant women but then proceeded to perform translumbar aortography (see page 23) on them. This was the first time that translumbar aortography had ever been done on pregnant women and its purpose was to study the abdominal circulation in advanced pregnancy.[1]

After the spinal anaesthetic, with consequent paralysis and loss of sensation of the lower limbs and trunk, the patients were turned to lie face downwards. A six-inch needle was then pushed through the mass of muscles adjacent to the vertebral column until it entered the aorta, the main artery of the body. When blood flowed in 'a pulsating stream' a contrast medium was injected through the needle and serial X-ray films were taken of the aorta and the renal arteries. The experiment was done on twelve women during the eighth month of pregnancy.

[1] Coutts, Opazo, Bianchi and Donoso, of Cuba, *American Journal of Obstetrics and Gynaecology*, 1935, **29**, 567.

One woman died of meningeal haemorrhage following the lumbar puncture given for the spinal anaesthetic.

The editor of the journal in which this experiment was reported appended a remarkable note to the article:

> This paper, contrary to our custom of not accepting contributions from foreign sources, is presented because of the unusual character of the daring experiment.

The word 'daring', which is certainly not out of place, signifies the taking of a major risk. But who ran this risk? Was it the patient, the doctors, or the unborn infant?

Thirteen years later the same procedure of translumbar aortography was done on sixty-eight women, all in the last stages of pregnancy, 'in order to investigate the possible value of aortography in the diagnosis of placenta praevia' (abnormal position of the afterbirth). In fact, only two of the subjects had this condition and none had any abnormality of heart, kidneys or blood pressure.

The procedure was as described previously, but with the addition that inflatable pressure cuffs were put on both thighs, so that the blood flow to the legs was greatly impeded. By this means, when the contrast medium was injected directly into the aorta it was prevented from entering the arteries of the legs, becoming concentrated in the abdominal arteries, and thus allowing better X-ray pictures. Incidentally, pressure cuffs applied in this way can readily produce syncope. When the X-rays had been completed the patients were given an infusion of three pints to combat shock (syncope).

As a result of the procedure two patients had high fever for a day. The report records that in thirteen of the patients the contrast medium was inadvertently injected outside the aorta instead of in it. But we are assured, 'except for pain in the lumbar region lasting twenty-four to forty-eight hours there were no ill effects'.[1]

In several other patients the contrast medium was accidentally injected into the main liver artery or into the coelic axis branch of the aorta; but in each of these cases without any apparent ill effect. The author records that the first time he

[1] Hartnett, of Firmin Disloge Hospital, St. Louis, *American Journal of Obstetrics and Gynaecology*, 1948, **55**, 940.

attempted this experiment on one of the above patients the entire contrast medium was injected by mistake into the left renal artery. He reports that no evidence of damage to the kidney of the patient to whom this happened could be observed up to four months after this incident. I would myself think that subsequent kidney damage could still have become manifest at a much later date. The author reports that in many of the patients labour began immediately after the aortic puncture and agrees that this was often not desirable. We are assured, 'all babies were living and apparently unaffected'.

An interesting experiment was conducted 'on women in various stages of pregnancy and with various complications' where the experimenters openly admit that their purpose bore no relation to the diagnosis or treatment of their subjects; it was solely to improve a technique they were developing – of visualising the circulation of the placenta.[1]

Twenty pregnant women were submitted to the following. A long wide-bore needle was inserted into the femoral artery immediately below the groin. Pneumatic cuffs were placed round the upper part of both thighs and inflated so as to occlude circulation to the legs. Through the needle a contrast medium was injected very rapidly (at the rate of sixteen milligrams per second) and under very high pressure (ninety pounds per square inch), and then serial X-rays were taken of the blood vessels of the uterus and placenta.

What is important is the statement made by the authors in their report that 'In this preliminary study no particular effort was made to select patients either for diagnosis or because they showed abnormalities, but rather to survey the possibilities of the technique as a diagnostic tool and as a research instrument for the study of placental circulation'.

This particular report is also interesting since it mentions – what is frequently omitted and what is very pertinent in pregnancy cases – the possible dangers of exposure to radiation (X-rays). 'In recent years', the authors wrote,

> the consequences of radiation exposure have become a major concern in Roentgenology and particularly where pregnant

[1] Solesh, Masterson and Hellman, of King's County Hospital, Brooklyn, New York, *American Journal of Obstetrics*, 1961, **81**, 57.

women are concerned. Keenly aware of this, we took every precaution to reduce radiation dosage to a minimum.

Why reduce to a minimum when there was no need to take X-rays at all? The authors add: 'Arteriography is not advocated as a routine procedure, but in indicated cases which present difficult diagnostic problems, this procedure may be of considerable value.' This kind of reasoning is unfortunately not uncommon. What it says is: We have done this experiment, which involves risk to the patient, without any cause to do so in terms of diagnosis or treatment – but we advise others not to, unless there is a definite diagnostic indication.

In 1963 some doctors set out to prove by experiment that the effect of the drug atropine on the heart and respiration of the foetus is identical with its effect on the heart and respiration of the adult.[1] The subjects chosen for this experiment were seven pregnant women, in three of whom labour had been induced by means of an intravenous infusion of the uterine stimulant oxytocin. A needle was pushed through the abdomen and into womb, and through this was passed a very fine platinum wire electrode. The electrode was made to enter the skin of the buttock of the foetus within the womb and from it recordings of the heart rate of the foetus were taken. (In one case the electrode was made to enter the scalp of the foetus.)

A second needle was then pushed through the patient's abdominal wall and into her womb. Through this a fine catheter was passed so that by means of it the pressures in the amniotic fluid (which surrounds the foetus) could be recorded on an electronic instrument. Thirdly, in order to record the patient's own blood pressure with more accuracy than is obtainable by the usual method, another catheter was placed in the femoral artery just below the groin, this catheter being connected with a recording instrument. Fourthly, an electrically recording thermometer was placed in the patient's rectum.

The drug atropine was then injected into the buttock of the foetus via the needle already inserted. While all this was going on the seven patients were in labour. The experimenters note

[1] Mendez-Bauer, Poseiro, Arrellano-Hernandez, Zambrana and Caldeyro-Barcia, of University of Uruguay, *American Journal of Obstetrics and Gynaecology*, 1963, **85,** 1033.

that puncture of the placenta, which would have resulted in serious haemorrhage, was avoided by 'radiological methods', but I am not sure what is meant by this. The report states that:

> There were no complications either to the mother or foetus. The infants are being followed up and no undesirable consequences of these studies have so far been observed.

In 1962 a doctor decided to test the effect of a certain drug on labour.[1] The drug used was Nialamide, which is a tranquilizer belonging to a group of compounds known chemically as mono-amine oxidase inhibitors, and it was given to a large number of pregnant women. A matter of special importance is that the report quotes an authoritative statement[2] describing the results of administering a *related* drug to pregnant mice and rabbits. The results on these animals were either interference with the pregnancy or haemorrhage into the placenta. No ill effects were detected in the women; the course of their labour was normal and so were the infants when they were born. But in view of the known effects on animals of a related drug, the undertaking seems to me to have involved an unjustifiable risk. Furthermore, an important and serious matter is the danger of what is technically known as potentiation, namely, that even up to two weeks after the patient has received nialamide serious reactions may result if that patient should be given morphia or pethidine. These drugs are often administered to patients during labour, and the effect, in such a case, would be as though a very large (i.e. toxic) dose had been given. This whole experiment seems to me to have been very ill conceived.

A hundred and fourteen women attending one hospital and a hundred and seventy attending another were given nialamide tablets during the last two weeks of their pregnancy. Equal numbers of pregnant women at the two hospitals were each given dummy tablets as controls. The physician does not mention whether the consent of those who were given nialamide was sought or, if it was, how it was sought and what the patients were told. Were they told anything or were they simply 'given' the tablets?

[1] S. L. Barron, of St. Thomas's and Lambeth Hospitals, London, *Journal of Obstetrics and Gynaecology*, 1962, **69**, 443.
[2] *Science*, 1960, **131**, 1101.

In 1963 an experiment was conducted of which the purpose was to measure blood pressures in the inferior vena cava in late pregnancy.[1] The subjects chosen were a series of women about to undergo Caesarean section. Pressures in the inferior vena cava were measured before the operation by means of a catheter and wire guide which were passed along the femoral vein. These pressures were recorded at various levels as the catheter was moved up the femoral vein as far as the right atrium of the heart. At each catheter position the doctors also measured the effects of changing the patient's posture from supine to lateral. The patients were then given a general anaesthetic and the pressure recordings were continued during the Caesarean operation. The pressure changes resulting from delivering the baby were also observed. In the case of two of the patients the pressures in the chorio-decidual space were also measured by means of inserting a needle through the uterine wall.

The patients now underwent Caesarean operation during which the catheters were kept in position. Before suture of the abdomen, the uterus was lifted forward by long stay sutures and a further injection of contrast medium was made. By this means the doctors were able to study inferior vena cava pressures when there could be no pressure from the uterus.

The finding was that in late pregnancy the inferior vena cava is partially obstructed when the patient is in a supine position and partially relieved when she is in a lateral position.

The precise degree of risk, to either mother or baby, in any of the above experiments, is, of course, not an easy thing to determine. But the reader will judge whether, apart from risk of actual harm, pregnant women should be used in any of the ways described. In most societies a pregnant woman is given special consideration because of her condition. Surely such regard should be more common, not less, in medical circles.

3. EXPERIMENTS ON MENTAL DEFECTIVES AND THE MENTALLY SICK

The use of a mental defective, or of a mentally ill person, as the subject of a medical experiment raises immediately the question

---

[1] D. B. Scott and M. G. Kerr, of Royal Infirmary, Edinburgh, *Journal of Obstetrics and Gynaecology* (British Commonwealth), 1963, **70,** 1044.

of consent in an acute form. We may ask two questions here, of which the second follows from the first. One: should such a person be regarded as *capable* of giving consent? He may be regarded in law as not wholly responsible for his acts towards others; is he to be so regarded in respect of what he may consent to have done to *him*? And to what extent can a mentally sick or defective subject understand the experimenter's explanation anyway? Two: should such subjects be used at all? I invite the reader to bear these questions in mind while looking at the following cases.

A group of workers wished to investigate some aspects of calcium metabolism and for this purpose chose ten mentally defective children who had no abnormality of calcium metabolism. They were given a radioactive compound by mouth and a month later the same substance by intravenous infusion.[1]

Another research worker, wishing to investigate iodine metabolism, chose as his subjects nineteen mentally defective children, who had no abnormality of iodine metabolism, and gave them a radioactive iodine compound.[2]

The same research worker gave radioactive thyroxine intravenously to a further seventeen mentally defective children who were free from any suspicion of thyroid diseases. This experiment necessitated obtaining daily blood samples for ten days.[3]

The following experiment was done on eighty elderly mental patients, the youngest of whom was sixty-six, but two were seventy-seven and one was eighty-four. Its purpose was to measure the brain blood flow in dementia. As controls five normal elderly patients (average age seventy-two), and nine mental patients (average age seventy-four) and eleven young medical students were used. Two long needles were each inserted deeply into each jugular vein, just below the angle of the jaw. A third needle was inserted into the femoral artery in the groin. When these needles were in position all 105 patients were made to inhale a radioactive gas through a tightly fitting

[1] Felix Bronner, Robert Harris, Maletskos and Benda, of Walter Fernold State School, Waverly, Mass., *Journal Clinical Investigation*, 1956, **35,** 78.

[2] Heskel M. Haddad, at District Columbia Training School, Laurel, Maryland, *Journal Pediatrics*, 1960, **57,** 391.

[3] Idem., *Journal Clinical Investigation*, 1960, **39,** 1590.

face mask. Four of the elderly control group were submitted to repeat studies.[1]

The blood flow to the brain was investigated in five patients with brain disease, one of whom had loss of speech and at least one other had mental impairment. Needles were inserted into their jugular veins and also into their femoral arteries. They inhaled a special gas mixture through a face mask. But after the control data had been established the patients were given an intravenous injection of a drug, tolbutamide, which has the effect of producing a marked fall of blood sugar. The tests were then repeated.[2] A low blood sugar may have serious consequences, especially in elderly people.

A similar type of experiment was carried out in 1953.[3] This time the subjects were four patients convalescing from a variety of diseases, about which the report gives no other details, and a further group which consisted of six schizophrenics. The purpose of the experiment was to study 'Changes in cerebral vascular resistance as a result of experimentally induced alkalosis and acidosis'.

Needles were inserted into both jugular veins and also into one femoral artery and the patients were then made to inhale a nitrous oxide mixture through tightly fitting face masks. After blood samples had been taken from the three needles, each of the patients was given an intravenous infusion of two pints of ammonium carbonate solution in order to produce alkalosis (excessive alkalinity of the blood). Further samples of blood were then taken. The patients now received intravenous infusions of a similar quantity of ammonium chloride so as to produce acidosis (excessive acidity of the blood). In other words, instead of waiting for patients to be admitted to hospital with conditions which produce alkalosis or acidosis, these toxic conditions were artificially induced in patients just so that their effects on brain circulation could be studied.

In 1962 a new antibiotic designed to treat acne vulgaris

[1] Lassen, Feinberg and Lane, of St. Elizabeth Hospital, Bethseda, Maryland, *Journal Clinical Investigation*, 1960, **39,** 491.

[2] Rosalie Burns, Ehrenreich, Alman and Fazekas, of New England Center Hospital, Boston, *American Journal of Medical Science*, 1961, **242,** 189.

[3] Schieve and W. P. Wilson, of Duke Hospital, Durham, N.C., and Butner State Hospital, *Journal of Clinical Investigation*, 1953, **32,** 33.

(pimples) was investigated.[1] The subjects, all of whom had acne, were fifty in number and were either juvenile delinquents or mental defectives. After oral administration of the drug for two weeks no fewer than 50% of the children were found to have sustained liver damage. In spite of this, however, the doctors continued to administer the drug with the expected result, that 'these liver abnormalities became more marked and in two children jaundice occurred'. In eight of the children subsequent liver punctures showed severe liver damage, and in four cases liver puncture was done at least twice. The report adds,

> Four of the patients were challenged with a 1g. dose of the drug after liver function had returned to normal. Within 1 or 2 days hepatic dysfunction again developed in 3 of the 4.

An anonymous author wrote wittily in the *British Medical Journal*:[2]

> Juvenile delinquency in U.S.A. seems to carry with it hazards not previously suspected. The pimpled gangster of to-day may find himself the bilious guinea pig of tomorrow. It seems a little hard, perhaps, for a boy who has spent his formative years learning how to dodge flick knives to fall a victim to intercostal perforation by a liver puncture needle.

An unusual experiment was done on a group of twenty-one mentally deficient or psychotic patients on whom lumbar punctures were performed and Tuberculin (a derivative from tubercle bacilli) was injected into the cerebrospinal fluid. The process was repeated daily for several days. It is recorded:[3]

> Ten hours after the injection the temperature begins to rise, pulse quickens, and a little later the patient usually vomits. The disturbance reaches its maximum about 24 hours after the injection. By this time the temperature is anything from 101 to 104 F, the patient is pale, listless, photophobic (profoundly disturbed by light) and reluctant to eat, while the neck is often a little stiff.

These symptoms lasted for two to three days, but the marked

---

[1] Tickton and H. J. Zimmerman, of Laurel's Children's Center, Maryland, *New England Journal of Medicine*, 1962, **267**, 964.
[2] *British Medical Journal*, 1962, **2**, 1536.
[3] J. Swithinbank, Honor Smith and Vollum, *Journal of Pathology*, 1953, **65**, 565.

changes in the cerebrospinal fluid produced lasted as long as three months. Stated differently, these patients had been given a meningitis.

Subsequently it was decided to compare these results with those obtained in twenty-five patients with Disseminated Sclerosis (three of whom were under eighteen). They also had lumbar punctures and injections of Tuberculin into their spinal canal. 'Twenty-four hours later and as often during the following fortnight as circumstances permitted', the same process, including the injection, was repeated.[1]

The report begins:

> It is now established that the injection of Tuberculin into the cerebrospinal fluid of a sensitized subject (one who has previously been given an identical injection) evokes a wave of inflammation involving the meninges (covering membranes) and the blood vessels of the brain and spinal cord.

It is reported that all the Disseminated Sclerosis patients gave their consent to the experiment after full explanation. But, concerning this consent, a doctor commented:[2]

> The patients with Disseminated Sclerosis were all volunteers, and you state that a control group of psychotics was used for comparison. Surely, I cannot be alone in finding this state of affairs disturbing? Even the experimental work with the diseased group may not be as permissible as it appears on the surface. Any patient with progressive incurable disease will submit to any procedure however hazardous, offered with whatever explanations and reservations. The pressure to volunteer is enormous, as I know with regret from past errors of my own in this respect. But allowing that the work is justifiable in this group, what are we to say about the psychotics who were submitted to an undertaking with considerable risk? Were they volunteers?

To this the authors replied:

> We sympathize with Mr. Le Vay's sentiments. It was considered that the transient pyrexia and cerebral hyperaemia

---

[1] Honor Smith, Espir, Whitty and Professor Ritchie-Russell, of United Oxford Hospital and Stoke Mandeville Hospital, Bucks., *Journal Neurology and Psychiatry*, 1957, **20**, 1.
[2] Le Vay, *Lancet*, 1957, **1**, 1040.

that accompanies the reaction might well be beneficial in mental disease . . . However the lack of volunteers is a constant hindrance to research work.[1]

The following experiment was carried out in 1961.[2] A child had been admitted to hospital with a severe illness (methaemoglobinaemia) caused by drinking contaminated well water. This was successfully treated by injecting a dye (methylene blue). The authors write:

In view of the paucity of reports on methylene blue overdosage and the prolonged cyanosis (blueness) and haemolytic anaemia (destruction of the red blood cells) resulting from such over-dose, it was felt that the purposeful duplication of the picture, if possible, would be of great value.

For this purpose a seven-day-old mentally defective infant was selected and the parents gave permission. The infant was injected with the dye and duly became blue. Then a further injection was given.

Soon afterwards the infant became markedly greyish in colour. . . . Occasional twitching was noticed and the infant fed poorly for several days. Otherwise the condition remained unchanged except for the ghastly colour.

But one week later, because of the destruction of its red blood corpuscles by the methylene blue, the infant developed an acute haemolytic anaemia, with jaundice from which it made a very slow recovery.

An extensive trial of an experimental measles vaccine was conducted in England and for this purpose fifty-six mentally subnormal children were selected.[3] The authors state, 'They were especially suitable for the study since close medical supervision was possible throughout.' Twenty-one other mental defectives were not vaccinated, but were kept in close contact with the vaccinated group.

[1] *Lancet*, 1957, **1**, 1057.
[2] Goluboff and Wheaton, of Saskatoon City Hospital, Saskatchewan, Canada, *Journal of Paediatrics*, 1961, **58**, 86.
[3] I. R. Aldous, B. H. Kerman and N. Butler, of Fountains Hospital, Tooting, London, and Queen Mary's Hospital, Carshalton, Surrey, *British Medical Journal*, 1961, **2**, 1250.

Forty-six of the vaccinated became feverish and forty-eight developed a rash. Twenty-two had a moderately severe and nine a very severe reaction to the vaccination. It is noted,

> Many of the vaccinated became miserable and fretful during the period of rash and pyrexia.

Five of the children developed tonsillitis as a consequence and one had a severe complicating broncho-pneumonia.

There is a report of another extensive use of an experimental measles vaccine carried out in Nigeria.[1]

A report of an experiment which evoked a great deal of comment was published in 1961.[2] This report described how three female mental defectives who had been found to have chromosome abnormalities in their blood were investigated. They were physically normal and had normal external sexual development. 'It was decided', wrote the physicians, 'to investigate the genital system of our patients as adequately as possible.' To do this the three girls were submitted to abdominal operations by means of which their ovaries could be examined and a piece removed for microscopic study. The conclusion arrived at by the experimenters was that all three girls were 'potentially fertile'.

Two of the comments made on this experiment are worth repeating here. The first is that of Dr. MacLean of University College Hospital, Nigeria, who wrote:

> If the inmates of homes for mental defectives, in America or elsewhere, are henceforward to be regarded as convenient material for the experimental surgeon, it is well that the public becomes aware of this dubious development in medical ethics.[3]

And the second is that of Dr. R. E. W. Fisher, who said:

> There is a terrible temptation for the researching physicians in the newly recognized chromosome anomalies. So many of the patients are mental defectives, so few come to post mortem, so much is being discovered so quickly. Nevertheless it is not within the ethics of our profession, or indeed of our civilization,

[1] P. Collard, Hendrickse, Montefiore, Sherman, van de Wall and D. Morley, of Wesley Guild Hospital, Ilasha, Nigeria, *British Medical Journal*, 1961, **2,** 1246.
[2] A. W. Johnston, Ferguson-Smith, Handmaker, H. W. Jones and G. S. Jones, of Johns Hopkins Hospital, Baltimore, *British Medical Journal*, 1961, **2,** 1046.
[3] *British Medical Journal*, 1961, **2,** 1645.

to forget that even these poor people are entitled to the rights of human beings.[1]

In order to study 'Factors influencing concentration gradients of protein in cerebrospinal fluid', the following experiment was done. As subjects twelve infants aged between one and nine months, all of whom were mentally deficient owing to hydrocephalus were chosen.[2] They were given an intravenous infusion of a radioactive compound. After that needles were inserted in three places: through the skull into the brain; though the back of the neck; and into the lumbar spine. From each of these sites specimens of cerebrospinal fluid were collected through the needles. The experiment was in no way connected with the treatment or investigation of hydrocephalus.

Whatever we may think about the special question of consent in the case of the mental defective and the mentally ill, I feel that the point hardly needs emphasizing, in the light of some of the examples cited in this chapter, that there is a wrong done to these unfortunate people when they are used as controls. If the subject of an experiment is incapable of giving or withholding a true consent – either because he cannot understand a medical explanation or because he is not really clear in his head about what he is doing – then he is a very easy subject to get hold of. If it is *no use* asking for his consent, then he can be used without being asked. It is impossible to resist the conclusion that this kind of reasoning is sometimes employed by experimenters. So far from the special consideration to which mental cases are entitled, some places discernibly choose the very opposite attitude. I have myself at times been shocked by students of my own who would favour the mass killing of psychotics. In support of their attitude (which would certainly be to allow the use of mental cases quite ruthlessly for experiments) they quote the words of the French-American doctor and Nobel prize winner, Alexis Carrel of The Rockefeller Institute, New York, who wrote:

> We have already referred to the vast sums at present spent upon the maintenance of prisons and lunatic asylums in order

---

[1] *British Medical Journal*, 1962, **1**, 112.
[2] R. A. Fishman, Ransohoff and Osserman, of Presbyterian and Francis Delafield Hospitals, New York, *Journal of Clinical Investigation*, 1958, **37**, 1419.

to protect the public from anti-social and insane persons. Why do we keep all these useless and dangerous creatures alive? . . . In Germany the Government has taken energetic measures against the multiplication of inferior types, the insane and criminals. The ideal solution would be to eliminate all such individuals as soon as they proved dangerous . . . Philosophic theory and sentimental prejudice are not entitled to a hearing in such a matter.[1]

If Dr. Carrel is right, then the use of mental cases as subjects for whatever experiment – however unrelated to the possible relief of their own condition – is automatically justified. If, however, the second is admissible, at what point on the road to 'elimination' do we call a halt?

4 · EXPERIMENTS ON PRISON INMATES

For many centuries the criminal has been regarded as an ideal subject on whom to perform medical experiments. Some of the ancient Persian kings allowed their physicians to use criminals as experimental material and the Ptolemys of Egypt adopted the same practice. In the sixteenth century the Grand Duke of Tuscany gave permission to Fallopius (after whom the Fallopian tubes connected with the womb are named) to use criminals for any experiments he liked. In the eighteenth century in England, Queen Caroline, wife of King George IV, when Princess of Wales, consented to her physician using six condemned criminals for experimental smallpox vaccination before submitting her own children to the procedure. Moreover, 'To make a further trial the Queen Caroline procured half a dozen of the charity children belonging to St. James' parish'.[2]

It is not, however, the ethics of 'donating' that we are concerned with in the present chapter but the use of the inmates of prisons as subjects for experiments by doctors engaged on research. The use of criminals as subjects for medical experiments is current practice in a number of American states; and since the subject of this book relates to medical practice in the West it will be relevant to our purpose to describe a number of instances from America.

[1] From *Man the Unknown* (Harpers, 1939).
[2] Sir Hans Sloane (Royal Physician), *Phil. Transactions of Britain*, 1755, **49**, 516.

Experiments on Prison Inmates

According to R. C. Fox,

It has been estimated that as many as twenty thousand Federal prisoners are participating as volunteers in medical experiments.[1]

The numbers are likely to have increased considerably since this was written in 1960.

Some of the German doctors on trial at Nuremberg in 1947 cited as part of their defence nine reports of experiments on criminals gathered from world medical literature. These, they claimed, were analogous to, and so justification of, their own activities. The following three American experiments were cited.

Professor Rose, who was indicted for using concentration-camp inmates for typhus experiments cited in his defence the work of Colonel Strong (later Professor of Tropical Medicine at Harvard). He had obtained the permission of the Governor of the Philippines, but without the knowledge of the victims, to infect with plague a group of criminals condemned to death. Later Colonel Strong produced beri-beri (a deficiency disease characterized by paralysis, mental disturbance and heart failure) in another group of Philippine convicts. One of these died as a result of the experiment.[2] It has been reported that the only reward given to the convicts was gifts of tobacco.

Professor Weltz, who had carried out large-scale experiments at Dachau referred to the work of Goldberger, who in 1915 made an unsuccessful attempt to discover a cure for pellagra. To do this he produced the disease, which is characterized by diarrhoea, dementia and dermatitis, in twelve white Mississippi convicts who became seriously ill as a consequence.[3] Before the experiment was made formal agreements were drawn up with the convicts' lawyers, agreeing to subsequent parole or release.

A third series of experiments quoted at that trial were conducted in 1944 in a Chicago prison and a New Jersey reformatory.[4] The convict volunteers were infected with malaria to try

[1] R. C. Fox, of Columbia University, New York, *Clinical Pharmacology and Therapeutics*, 1960, **1**, 423.
[2] *Philadelphia Journal of Science*, 1906, **1**, 1512.
[3] *Public Health Reports*, 1915, **30**, 3336.
[4] Ralph Jones, Craige, Alving, C. M. Whorton, Pulmann and Lillian Eithelberger, in Stateville Penitentiary, Chicago, and Berliner, D. Pearle, Taggar, Zubrod, J. Welch, Conan, Bauman, Scudder and J. A. Shannon, in New Jersey State Reformatory, Special Supplement to *Journal Clinical Investigation*, 1948.

out new cures. At Stateville Penitentiary 441 convicts were used. I have not been able to ascertain the figures for the experiment at New Jersey State Reformatory, but from the reports they would appear to have been almost equally large. A lengthy notice was posted in Stateville prison describing in detail the nature of the tests and the risks. All were required to sign the following document:

> I . . ., No. . . . aged . . ., hereby declare that I have read and clearly understood the above notice, as testified by my signature hereon, and I hereby apply to the University of Chicago, which is at present engaged on malarial research at the orders of the Government, for participation in the investigations of the life-cycle of the malarial parasite. I hereby accept all risks connected with the experiment and on behalf of my heirs and my personal and legal representatives I hereby absolve from such liability the University of Chicago and all the technicians and assistants taking part in the above-mentioned investigations. I similarly absolve the Government of the State of Illinois, the Director of the Department of Public Security of the State of Illinois, the warden of the State Penitentiary at Joliet-Stateville and all employees of the above institutions and Departments, from all responsibility, as well as from all claims and proceedings or Equity pleas, for any injury or malady, fatal or otherwise, which may ensue from these experiments.
>
> I hereby certify that this offer is made voluntarily and without compulsion. I have been instructed that if my offer is accepted I shall be entitled to remuneration amounting to . . . dollars, payable as provided in the above Notice.

The published account of these experiments states:

> Since in these studies drugs were administered in doses approaching the estimated maximum tolerated dose, toxicity was expected and found.

Many of the patients became profoundly ill because of the malarial infection which had been induced in them. Many of them suffered from the toxic effects of the experimental drugs used to treat their induced malaria, including abdominal pain which was often severe, loss of appetite, nausea, vomiting, cyanosis (blueness), transient changes in their electrocardiograms, drug fever, skin lesions and marked fall of blood pressure.

Experiments on Prison Inmates

That special considerations are involved in the use of prison inmates as subjects for medical experiments was acknowledged by a special tribunal appointed by Governor Green of Illinois in 1948 to examine the problem.[1] This committee recommended, amongst other things:

(a) That the subjects must be volunteers informed of the possible hazards. 'Volunteering exists when a person is able to say "yes" or "no" without fear of being punished or of being deprived of privileges due to him in the ordinary course of events.

(b) 'The choice of volunteers must be made on the basis of established criteria.'

(c) That prior animal experiments must have been undertaken.

(d) That all unnecessary injury and physical and mental suffering be avoided.

The Green committee was principally concerned with rewards and on this problem expressed the following opinions:

The reduction of sentence in prison under the parole system is viewed as a reward for good conduct. Service as a subject in a medical experiment is considered to be a form of good conduct. . . . The extent to which the service of a prisoner in an experiment is motivated by good social consciousness on the one hand and by the desire for a reduction of sentence in prison on the other is a matter for consideration in the case of each prisoner. . . .

A reduction of sentence in prison, if excessive or drastic, can amount to undue influence. If the sole motive of the prisoner is to contribute to human welfare, any reduction in sentence would be a reward. If the sole motive of the prisoner is to obtain a reduction in sentence, an excessive reduction in sentence which would exercise undue influence in obtaining consent of prisoners would be inconsistent with the principle of voluntary participation.

The woolliness of many of these opinions is in some measure an indication of the difficulties inherent in the problems which the committee set out to solve, but often evaded. Thus, the

[1] Full report was published in *Journal American Medical Association*, 1948, **136,** 457.

63

extent to which a prisoner's volunteering is motivated by 'good social consciousness' is something impossible to determine and the recommendation that volunteers should be chosen on the basis of 'established criteria' is virtually meaningless.

In fact, the ethical problems associated with the use of prison inmates as subjects for medical experiments are largely of artificial creation, because the basic problem of the essential purpose of prisons and punishments has not been solved. Society has enough difficulties in dealing effectively, constructively and humanely with its prisoners without complicating the issues still further with rewards for volunteering for experiments.

As long ago as 1856 the use of criminals in experimental medicine was condemned outright by Claude Bernard in his famous book on the subject. And as recently as 1961 the World Medical Association urged that 'persons retained in prisons, penitentiaries or reformatories, being captive groups, should not be used as the subjects of experiments'.[1]

This recommendation of the World Medical Association has not, however, been formally adopted by that organization. As 'Pertinax' in the *British Medical Journal* for January 1963 wrote:

> I am disturbed that the World Medical Association is now hedging on its clause about using criminals as experimental material. The American influence has been at work on its suspension. I am surprised at this. The Americans were the first in the field to apply to human experimentation the ghastly lessons of the Nuremberg trial. Now they have forgotten that the Nazi doctors regarded the inhabitants of Auschwitz as criminals and did not hesitate to experiment on them. Of course I know there are differences. Profound differences. There was the bestial and sadistic element in so many of the German experiments. The Americans take great pains to obtain consent. But the Nuremberg code, guide to so much of what was subsequently adopted in America, expressly warns against experimenting on captive populations. One of the nicest American scientists I know was heard to say: 'Criminals in our penitentiaries are fine experimental material – and much cheaper than chimpanzees.' I hope the chimpanzees don't come to hear of this.

Indeed, so far from doctors implementing in practice the World

[1] *British Medical Journal*, 1962, **2**, 1119.

Experiments on Prison Inmates

Medical Association's recommendation that 'captive groups' should not be used as experimental subjects, recent reports indicate that this particular kind of subject is being used, in America, more and more. In July 1963 *Time* magazine cited the following cases in the course of a survey of the use of prisoners:

1. An inmate of the Mississippi State Penitentiary at Pachman who was serving a life sentence for murder developed cancer of the lung. He was transferred to the University Medical Center at Jackson. His diseased lung was removed and he received the transplant of the lung of a patient who had recently died from a heart attack. The operation was not successful and the man died two weeks later.

2. The *Time* article stated that the Federal Government sponsored medical research in fifteen out of thirty-seven penal institutions, some of the biggest projects having been undertaken in the U.S. Penitentiary in Atlanta. In return for submitting to experiments, federal prisoners get rewards ranging from a packet of cigarettes to twenty-five dollars in cash. If an experiment is particularly onerous or carries some risk of major discomfort the Bureau of Prisoners may give the prisoner 'meritorious good time credits', which 'shave a few days off his sentence'.

3. Apart from the Federal system at least a dozen states allow prisoners to be recruited for research experiments. Thus the Ohio State Penitentiary in Columbus has provided volunteers for cancer research experiments. These men were given injections of live cancer cells. (None of them developed cancer.) At Cook County jail in Chicago prisoner-volunteers were injected with blood from patients who had leukemia. (None of these contracted the disease either.) What is important, however, is the purpose of the experiment, which was to see whether either disease could be transmitted to others. *Before* these experiments the possibility that they could have been was quite definite.

4. In Oklahoma State Penitentiary it was found that the medical director had made deals with pharmaceutical companies to test out their new drugs on prisoners. For volunteering as subject for these tests the prisoners received small fees. The doctors grossed an estimated three hundred thousand dollars a year.

5. A more ambitious and financially even more rewarding programme was undertaken by these same doctors by means of which prisoners could donate their blood – or rather sell it – so that the doctors could then, so to speak, retail it. The success of this scheme was due to the recent finding that a man can donate blood as often as once a week (instead of only two or three times a year as had been the previous limit), provided only that the plasma is kept and the blood cells themselves are promptly re-infused into the donor. Under this scheme the prisoners received five dollars per quart while the two doctors sold the blood at fifteen dollars per quart. While agreeing that the receipt of the money and the help to the prisoners' self-respect because thay had given their blood were both good for morale, state officials decided that such a scheme should not be operated for private profit. It is therefore being turned over to a research council headed by medical professors.

In 1963 an interesting account appeared in the medical press of an experiment performed on volunteers from the Kansas State Penitentiary.[1] Originally eighty-four men aged between forty and sixty-five volunteered. Thirty-two of these were disqualified because they were found to have positive signs in their cardiovascular or nervous systems, or abnormal changes in the electrical tracings from their brains. Six changed their minds and declined 'for personal reasons'. For technical reasons three others had to be left out. The experiment was thus finally carried out on forty-three men, of whom thirty-six were Caucasians and seven were negroes.

The procedure was as follows. A needle was inserted into a brachial artery and a wire guide and catheter passed through the needle so as to enter the ascending aorta. A contrast medium was then injected through the catheter and serial X-rays taken to study the brain (and also, incidentally, the renal) circulation. There were no complications. Permission for this experiment was granted by the Chancellor of the University of Kansas, by the Board of Regents and the Director of Penal Institutions, and by the Attorney-General of the State of Kansas. The experiment was conducted by Dr. Faris and associates,

[1] Faris, Poser, O. W. Wilmore and C. H. Agnew, of University Medical Center, Kansas City, *Neurology*, 1963, **13**, 386.

66

who, in their report, 'wish to express our appreciation to the inmates of Kansas State Penitentiary, without whose generous co-operation the study would not have been possible'.

In a recent issue of *Medical News*[1] it is reported that at Holmsburg Prison (a federal prison in Pennsylvania) nine out of every ten prisoners volunteer as subjects for medical experiments and that this volunteering is done in spite of the fact that the prisoners are warned that the experiments may cause them discomfort or pain. This prison has cells specially equipped for medical research and two of the prisoners have been trained as technicians. The volunteers are used in tests to determine the effects on the human body of new chemical products, drugs, and of new medical techniques. According to this article, several thousand men in United States prisons are currently undergoing such tests. The prison authorities 'donate' the time of their inmates and the space needed for the work. In most prisons the research organization in charge of the tests pays the convicts for volunteering. As the convicts have almost identical diets, sleeping hours and daily routine, they provide a most convenient set of subjects for controlled clinical trials.

An American lawyer has expressed the opinion:

> Prison experiments should not involve any promise of parole or of commutation of sentence; this would be what is called in the law of confessions, undue influence or duress through promise of reward, which can be as effective in overbearing the will as threats of harm. Nor should there be pressure to conform within the prison generated by the pattern of rejecting parole application of those who do not participate. It should not be made informally a condition of parole that one be a good prisoner and subject himself to medical experimentation.[2]

When considering the whole question of experiments on convicts it must not be forgotten that the status of 'criminal' can be thrust upon innocent people. Many Nazi doctors justified their experiments by designating all the inmates of concentration camps, 'criminals'.

The cases quoted in this chapter have all been, as I mentioned, from America. Although, so far as I know, there are no

[1] *Medical News*, 12 March 1964.
[2] Professor F. A. Freund in Gay Lecture, Harvard Law School, *New England Journal of Medicine*, 1965, **273**, 687.

such cases on recent record in Great Britain, there is no great ground for British complacency on this point. For we have evidence of a clear desire on the part of some experimenters to use criminals in this way. Quite recently, Dr. W. P. Kennedy, Principal Medical Officer of the Distillers' Company, wrote recommending the use of criminals to test drug toxicity, and went on:

> It is said that public opinion would never accept such a ruling in Britain, but it is difficult to see why not.[1]

It is my hope that the reader will understand 'why not' and will not lend his support to any movement which would make, of the British prison inmate, one more category of abused persons.

5. EXPERIMENTS ON THE DYING AND THE OLD

It is difficult to write objectively and unemotionally about experiments performed on very old people or those who are dying, but the reader can form his own judgments concerning the experiments quoted in this section.

About 1950 a new technique was evolved for the investigation of patients with liver disease. This consisted in thrusting a needle into the spleen to a depth of about three inches, so as to measure the blood pressure in the splenic veins, this being an index of the pressure in the liver veins. Furthermore, by injecting a contrast medium through the needle, X-ray pictures can be obtained of the splenic and liver circulation. This procedure, called percutaneous splenoportography, was further developed in 1955, when three patients with advanced cancer were used. Having thereby achieved the necessary technical skill, the experiment was then repeated forty times on thirty-two patients, seven of whom had cirrhosis of the liver, two had extra-hepatic venous occlusion, three had benign abdominal swellings. No details of the other seventeen patients are given. Concerning the patients with advanced cancer the authors admit:

> The splenoportograms in these patients were of little direct value except to enlarge our appreciation of the effects of advanced cancers.

[1] *The Practitioner* (London), 1963, **190**, 9.

They remark, 'When carried out properly it seldom causes more than modest pain'. In their summary they comment:[1]

The procedure is technically simple, generally successful, seldom seriously discomforting to the patients, and reasonably safe.

Yet they record that the injection usually caused flushing, nausea and headache and that two patients had very severe pain because of the accidental injection of the contrast medium into either the pleural or peritoneal cavity instead of into the spleen. One of these patients required 'an exploration a few days later', which means an abdominal operation to find out what damage, if any, had resulted. What do the experimenters mean by the epithets, 'seldom', 'reasonable' and 'modest'? A further interesting comment, which incidentally applies to many experiments described in this book, is:

Our experience and those of others suggests that rare catastrophic reactions to an injection of a radiographic contrast materials cannot be predicted.

Another method of portal venography was developed on fourteen patients with advanced cancer who had a short life expectancy.[2] A six-inch needle was inserted through the abdomen into a main liver vein so as to measure the pressure in that vein and to collect blood samples from it. In addition some of the patients had an injection through the needle of a contrast medium so that serial X-rays could be taken.

A further paper records the repetition of this experiment.[3] In this series, however, all the patients had contrast medium injected into their livers and serial X-rays taken. The authors explain that, having developed the technique on a number of corpses, they then proceeded to practise it on thirty-five patients 'with short life expectancy because of cancer'. They also obtained, in addition, 'satisfactory' pictures from two

[1] M. Figley, W. J. Fry, Orebaugh and H. M. Pollard, of Ann Arbor, Michigan, *Gastroenterology*, 1955, **28**, 153.
[2] H. R. Bierman, Steinbach, L. P. White and K. H. Kelly, of University of California School of Medicine, *Proceedings Society Experimental Medicine and Biology*, 1952, **79**, 550.
[3] Steinbach, H. R. Bierman, E. R. Miller and Wass, of University of California School of Medicine, *Radiology*, 1953, **60**, 368.

patients who had neither cancer nor liver disease (about whom no further details are given), and from four patients suffering from advanced liver cirrhosis. The report records that on most occasions a small amount of the contrast medium escaped outside the portal vein, but with 'no obvious ill effects'. In the case of one patient the contrast medium was accidentally injected into the liver cells themselves. The immediate result of this was considerable pain which lasted for three days. From an accident of this kind, however, serious and permanent damage could result later on.

Another similar experiment was conducted on patients with advanced cancer.[1] On this occasion hollow needles six inches in length were deeply inserted directly into the patients' livers and catheters were then passed through the needles so as to enter a hepatic or portal vein. Blood samples were then taken and a contrast medium injected, after which X-rays of the liver circulation were taken.

In fourteen of the patients who were studied in this way the catheter was kept in the liver for periods ranging from two to *nineteen days* so that frequent and numerous blood samples from the liver could be taken. This experiment was carried out twice on each of seventy-three patients described as 'severely ill', but about whom there is very little other information except that, 'Since many of the patients studied had widespread neoplastic disease (cancer) it was possible to follow most of them until their death.' The difficulty of the technique may be gauged from the fact that on one patient who had multiple nerve tumours five unsuccessful attempts were made. Out of the total of seventy-three patients, only in the case of two, who had cirrhosis of the liver, could the experiment be said to have direct relevance.

The authors somewhat surprisingly record that, 'There were no serious complications. Several unexpected findings were encountered'. They mention, however, that in three patients the needle accidentally pierced the bowel; in two instances it punctured a main artery; another patient had his gall bladder punctured; one patient had syncope (shock); and three had

[1] H. R. Bierman, L. P. White, K. H. Kelly, Coblentz and A. Fisher, of the University of California Medical School, *Journal of the American Medical Association*, 1955, **158**, 1331.

large haemorrhages. One wonders in what sense the phrase, 'not serious' is used.

In 1951 an elaborate experiment was conducted of which the essential aim was the development of a new technique, the passage of a catheter along a main artery, against the blood stream. The subjects were twenty-four patients with advanced cancer, including a child of eight with cancer of the tonsil, another child of eight with a tumour of the eye, and an infant of fourteen months with a malignant abdominal tumour. These children had anaesthetics, but the others did not. The authors state:[1]

> The procedure, including its hazards, and risks and its experimental nature, was explained to each patient, and an unqualified agreement was obtained in all cases.

The experimenters were able to demonstrate that it is possible under X-ray control to pass such a catheter through the brachial, femoral or carotid (neck) artery, which had been exposed by a long skin incision, into such remote arteries as those supplying the intestine, the thyroid gland in the neck, the stomach, the spleen, the spinal cord, the breast and the buttocks.

One patient developed an infection from the incision and had a severe haemorrhage from it. Another patient, who had cancer and also high blood pressure and heart involvement, had a stroke five minutes after the procedure had started and died four days later.

In a third patient, 'The physician became confused in the dark of the X-ray room and accidentally twisted the carotid artery into a knot.' As a consequence of this, the patient suffered a stroke twelve hours later. In a fourth patient, described as 'moribund', thrombosis of a main artery occurred, and this patient died forty-eight hours after the investigation.

The experimenters' comments concerning these events are revealing. They wrote:

> While four serious complications would appear to give a high incidence, it is not prohibitively high considering the initial effort in this direction, mostly on critically ill patients. New techniques encounter difficulties until they are perfected.

[1] H. R. Bierman, E. R. Miller, K. S. Dod, K. H. Kelly, R. L. Byron and D. H. Black, University of California Medical School, *American Journal Roentgenology*, 1951, **66,** 555.

What is Being Done

In 1953 another new technique was tried out.[1] The subjects on this occasion were ten patients all of whom had advanced malignant disease and all of whom are described in the report as having been volunteers. The procedure consisted in making an incision above the collar-bone and passing a catheter, or very wide needle, into the thoracic duct, which is the main channel draining the lymph from the body into a main vein of the chest. In the case of five of the ten subjects a contrast medium was injected into the duct and serial X-ray photographs were taken. In all ten subjects the catheter or needle was left in position, that is, in the subject, for from three to ten days. The amount of lymph drained away was consequently enormous (between one and five pints *per day*). To replace this huge loss it was necessary to give the subjects large transfusions of blood or plasma. The report states: 'There were no beneficial or deleterious effects of the procedure.'

A similar procedure of insertion of a catheter into the thoracic duct was done by another research team on four patients with advanced cancer. In these patients, however, an additional investigation was examination of the lymph in the thoracic duct after the oral administration of two different radioactive compounds. In these patients also infusions had to be given intravenously to make up for the large volumes of fluid lost by drainage of the lymph.[2]

In 1950 a group of doctors described the development of the technique known as retrograde cardiac catheterization for radiological visualization of the main branches of the thoracic aorta, including the coronary arteries. By this method a catheter over a yard long is passed, under X-ray control, against the blood stream via a main limb artery as far as the left ventricle. This is more difficult and hazardous than the usual method of cardiac catheterization via a limb vein and into the right side of the heart. To pass the catheter the main artery of the thigh or arm was exposed through an incision and the artery itself was incised so that the catheter could be passed into it. A contrast medium was then injected through the catheter and serial

[1] H. R. Bierman, R. L. Byron, K. H. Kelly, Gilfillian, L. P. White, N. E. Freeman and Petrakis, of University of California Medical School, San Francisco, *Journal of Clinical Investigation*, 1953, **32**, 637.

[2] Leon Hellman, Fazell and R. S. Rosenfield, of Memorial Hospital, New York, *Journal of Clinical Investigation*, 1960, **39**, 1288.

X-rays taken. After the experiment was completed the artery and the limb wound had to be repaired by stitching. But in some patients repair of the artery was found to be impossible, and the artery had to be tied and cut across completely. This will have the effect of grossly diminishing the blood supply to the limb.

The authors themselves state, 'The present study was basically experimental.' It was performed on twenty-four patients. One of these was a woman aged eighty-eight who was comatose as a result of a stroke. The contrast medium was injected no fewer than five times into the region of her aortic valve and serial X-rays taken after each injection. Immediately after the fifth injection she died.[1]

Another subject was a man of seventy-four dying from the fatal disease of myelomatosis. At the time of the experiment he is described as having been 'obviously moribund and deeply comatose'. This man received six injections of the contrast medium into his aorta and died six hours after the last one. 'The procedure', comment the experimenters, 'was probably not at fault.'

Another patient, aged sixty-six, had a large cancer of the chest; a fourth was a girl suffering from congenital heart disease. A fifth subject was a woman of twenty-four who was semi-conscious following a head injury. The report on this patient says:

> After a second injection of the contrast medium this patient became very excited at this point, but soon quieted. Because the brachial artery had been damaged during the period of excitement it was considered advisable to ligate it (tie it up). No sequelae developed . . . The patient was discharged later, completely recovered.

A study of heart output in twenty-one patients with severe anaemia has been described.[2] For this study cardiac catheterization was carried out. Among the patients was a woman of seventy-seven with a very severe anaemia (haemoglobin being only 22% of normal – see page 45), due to cancer of her bladder.

[1] Helmsworth, J. McGuire and Felson, of Cincinnati General Hospital, *American Journal Roentgenology*, 1950, **64**, 196.
[2] Sharpey-Schaffer, at Hammersmith Hospital, London, *Clinical Science*, 1945, **5**, 125.

Another was a woman of seventy-seven with a haemoglobin of only 14% of normal, due to pernicious anaemia. Another patient was a man of eighty-four with a haemoglobin of 30% due to intestinal haemorrhage.

In order 'to see if glycerol can be given safely to humans intravenously', after preliminary testing on animals, this substance was given by an intravenous infusion lasting three to six hours, to a group of twelve patients with cancer, whose life expectancy was deemed to be short. The patients included one woman of seventy-three and two of seventy-five.[1]

By accident a woman patient was given an intravenous infusion of sterile water instead of a different infusion. This resulted in severe destruction of her red blood corpuscles, and this in its turn caused acute kidney failure. This patient, however, fortunately recovered without sustaining 'any known renal damage'. The authors state:[2]

> Intravenous haemolysis (destruction of red blood corpuscles) of moderate or severe degree in man is often followed by acute renal failure. . . . The present studies were made to clarify this picture.

So, on the basis of this accident, which only by chance was not fatal, the doctors decided to investigate the earliest phases of anuria (suppression of kidney function). To do this they deliberately produced the anuria by intravenous administration of a large volume of water over a period of many hours. They used nine patients who were receiving X-ray treatment for leukemia, lymphadenoma or lymphosarcoma, all malignant fatal conditions. This caused the expected destruction of their red blood cells, which in turn brought about the renal failure which the doctors wished to investigate. The investigators state, 'The resultant alteration in renal function returned toward normal after the infusion of water had been discontinued or after the intravenous injection of parathormone.'

The renal function tests necessitated the infusion of inulin or diodrast into the vein of one leg and glucose solution alternating with the sterile water into the vein of the other leg. All the

[1] Sloviter and Rita Tietze of University Pennsylvania, Philadelphia, *Journal of Clinical Investigation*, 1958, **37**, 619.

[2] C. R. B. Blackburn, Hensley, Grant and F. B. Wright, of Albert Memorial Hospital, Sydney, Australia, *Journal of Clinical Investigation*, 1954, **33**, 825.

patients had catheters inserted into their bladders. The physicians inform us that 'some patients without malignant disease were studied after this experimental procedure proved harmless'. But actually the report gives particulars of only one such patient, who is described as 'neurasthenic'.

A report was published in 1963 describing an experiment concerning 'Oxygen consumption in paralysed men exposed to cold'. Three subjects were chosen: a patient aged thirty-four with polio who was paralysed from the neck down and whose breathing was kept going by a respirator; an unconscious patient aged sixty-eight who had been in that condition for three months following an abdominal operation (done elsewhere), complicated by shock with fall of blood pressure and resultant brain damage, and who was also being kept alive by means of a respirator; and an unconscious patient of seventeen who had been in that condition for twelve months as a result of severe head injuries for whom no respirator was necessary.[1]

The basal metabolic rate of the first of these subjects was studied without the use of drugs and then again while he was receiving a dose of tubocurarine (a drug which causes paralysis of muscles, including the respiratory muscles). All these subjects were made to breathe oxygen through a closed circuit apparatus and also received amounts of tubocurarine. Observations were made for forty minutes while the subjects were recumbent and covered with blankets. The blankets were then removed and fans played cool air over them for eighty to two hundred and ten minutes, during which periods the observations were continued. The subjects were then covered again with blankets and warmed with a 'heat cradle' and the observations repeated. Temperatures were taken in the mouth, on the skin and in the oesophagus (the last by means of passing a tube into the patient's gullet).

A new method of measuring the blood flow of the collateral veins of the liver has been described.[2] According to the published report the safety of the technique, which had included the use of a radioactive compound, had been established by a

[1] R. H. Johnson, A. C. Smith and Spalding, of United Oxford Hospitals, *Journal of Physiology*, 1963, **169**, 584.
[2] Iber, D. N. S. Kerr, Dolle and Sheila Sherlock, of Hammersmith Hospital London, *Journal of Clinical Investigation*, 1960, **39**, 1201.

preliminary testing which involved injecting this substance directly into the spleen of eight patients who had very large spleens, apparently without ill effects.

For the present experiment twelve patients were chosen. Of these seven had liver disease, three had severe diseases of the blood (thalasaemia and myelofibrosis), one had sarcoid and one Hodgkin's disease. Myelofibrosis and Hodgkin's disease are both fatal conditions and the investigation to which these two patients were submitted had no relation whatever to these diseases.

First, the patients were submitted to hepatic vein catheterization, a catheter being passed through an arm vein into and through the heart chambers and so into the liver vein. Second, a cannula was inserted into the femoral artery of the thigh. Third, a dye was infused[1] into an arm vein. Fourth, a large needle was inserted into the spleen, and through this a radioactive substance was 'deeply injected into the spleen'. Pressures within the spleen were measured before and after the injection. Blood samples were removed from the femoral and from the hepatic vein every five seconds during five minutes and a further single sample was taken from each at the end of ten minutes, i.e. at least 122 blood samples were taken from each patient.

Elderly people were used in an experiment to determine the total volume of blood in the thorax.[2] The doctors studied three groups of subjects. The first group were ten patients with mitral stenosis (valvular disease) who had cardiac failure. The second group were a control series of thirteen other patients who had heart failure from other causes including coronary disease. Among these were four patients over seventy and one over eighty. The third group were a further control series of ten other patients, including a man of seventy-four, all of whom were free from any disease of the cardiovascular system.

The procedure consisted of cardiac catheterization with the injection of a dye through an arm vein'. A large needle was kept in a main artery in order to take blood samples. Most of the

---

[1] Infusion of a dye is not the same procedure as the injection of a contrast medium for radiology. Dyes are infused into the circulation so that blood samples can be obtained later which will give some indication of the efficiency of a particular organ by assessing the extent to which the dye has been concentrated or absorbed.

[2] Kopelman and G. de J. Lee, of Hammersmith Hospital, London, *Clinical Science*, 1951, **10**, 383.

patients with heart failure were studied twice (before and after improvement of their condition).

In 1961 an experimental technique was tried out by which it was hoped to show enlarged glands in the chest.[1] For this investigation fifty-one patients were chosen who had cancer, two others who had heart failure and a further three who had cirrhosis of the liver. The doctors also used eleven 'normal controls' about whom no details are given.

Under local anaesthetic a needle was inserted into a rib and 'slowly and carefully driven with a small mallet' until the needle entered the bone marrow. When this had been done a contrast medium was rapidly injected through the needle and serial X-ray photographs were taken to outline the azygos veins of the chest, and possibly thereby to show up any enlarged glands.

Diabetic coma is a very serious condition with a high mortality. The longer the patient has been in coma prior to its energetic treatment the worse the outlook. This condition is associated with a profound fall of blood pressure. In order therefore to investigate the mechanism by which this fall comes about, it was decided by a group of research workers to pass cardiac catheters for special estimations on a group of patients admitted in diabetic coma. Oxygen consumption was also measured by a special apparatus.

This was done on five such patients, whose period of coma prior to admission varied between five and eighteen hours. One of these patients was aged seventy-one. All died, not because of this investigation, but because of the seriousness of the condition. I find it impossible to justify such a procedure which was purely experimental and very unlikely to have been of the slightest value to any of those particular patients.[2]

Concerning all the experiments described in this section it appears that doctors sometimes forget that those who are in most need of help, sympathy and gentle treatment are not the less sick but the most sick, and that among these the dying and the old have pre-eminent claims. Yet such subjects are often

---

[1] Bachman, Ackerman and Macken, of Frances Delafield Hospital, New York, *Annals of Surgery*, 1961, **153**, 344.
[2] Sheila Howarth, J. McMichael and Sharpey-Schafer, of Hammersmith Hospital, London, *Clinical Science*, 1948, **6**, 247.

included to provide an extra control series, or as subjects for experiments in which the doctors are still teaching themselves new techniques which 'encounter difficulties until they are perfected'.[1]

As Dr. Guttentag has written:

> Experimentation on the hopelessly sick requires a terrific amount of self-criticism, self-discipline, and understanding of life's essential attributes, lest it be perverted to unconscious barbarity.[2]

I am in complete agreement with Professor Beecher, who has written:[3]

> My deep conviction is that those who are in imminent danger of death should not be subjected to experimentation, except as part of the therapeutic effort for the benefit of the subject himself. Occasional reports are found wherein use of the 'hopelessly incurable' seems to justify dangerous experimentation. The error in this appears evident. It is not the physician's prerogative to make or to profit from such dubious judgements.

6. EXPERIMENTS ON THE EXPERIMENTERS THEM-SELVES

There are many recorded examples of experiments being performed by doctors on themselves. The distinguished English surgeon John Hunter in 1767, in order to prove that gonorrhoea is a transmissible disease inoculated himself with pus taken from a patient with gonorrhoea. But at the same time he inoculated himself accidentally with syphilis, from which infection he suffered dire consequences in later years. Purkinje, the Bohemian neuro-physiologist, deliberately took nine times the known toxic dose of digitalis for a cat. Digitalis is a drug with a powerful heart action. As a result he became seriously ill and vomited almost continuously for a week. An English physician, Hales, famous for his work on the circulation of blood, in his enthusiasm for the newly discovered intravenous route for medication, per-

---

[1] See page 71.

[2] O. E. Guttentag, of University School of Medicine, California, *Science*, 1953, 117, 207.

[3] H. K. Beecher, Massachusetts General Hospital, Boston, Mass., *Clinical Investigation in Medicine* (Legal, ethical and moral aspects), edited by I. Ladimer amd R. W. Newman, Boston University Research Institute Publication, 1963.

suaded a friend to inject half an ounce of castor oil into one of his (Hales's) veins. This proved almost fatal. In 1910 Pierre Curie, when told that radium could produce skin burns, bandaged some radium on to his own forearm and allowed it to remain for several hours, a severe burn resulting.

All these experiments could justifiably be described as foolhardy. But had they been done on patients they would have merited stronger criticism.

Many medical-research workers when questioned express a willingness to be the subject of some particular experiment, but it cannot be emphasized too strongly that ultimate proof of that willingness is the actual submission to the whole of the experiment under discussion and not merely to part of it. In order to establish his good faith it is not sufficient for an experimenter to allow himself to be submitted to only a part of some complex experiment, especially if it is the most innocuous part of the procedure. For example, a physician may claim that cardiac catheterization is harmless, and may support the contention by submitting himself to the investigation. But he cannot consider that this is justification for performing, not simple catheterization of the right side of the heart, but combined right- and left-sided heart catheterization, probably with some additional embellishment, such as the poking of a needle through the chest direct into a heart chamber. Furthermore, it is important to remember that the complex experiment is likely to be done on a sick patient, not a healthy volunteer like the experimenter himself. The willingness of a physician to experiment on himself never constitutes a complete justification for repeating the experiment on patients.

It is certainly a good thing that an experimenter should sometimes submit himself to exactly the same experiments as those which he intends to conduct on others. As Sir George Pickering, Professor of Medicine at Oxford, remarked in his presidential address to the Royal Society of Medicine in 1949:

> The experimenter has one golden rule to guide him as to whether the experiment is justifiable. Is he prepared to submit himself to the procedure? If he is, and if the experiment is actually carried out on himself, then it is probably justifiable. If he is not, then the experiment should not be done.[1]

[1] *Proceedings of the Royal Society of Medicine*, 1949, **42**, 231.

But the fact that the experimenter may be prepared to submit to a particular experiment, though good in itself, is not a *complete* justification for his carrying out that experiment on a layman. Self-experimentation cannot be regarded as the ultimate criterion of what is and what is not permissible for a doctor to impose on a patient or on any volunteer. Some people deliberately expose themselves to stupid risks, whether these be driving cars or experimenting on themselves. But this does not entitle them to expose others to these risks or to make others submit to their folly. A professor of clinical medicine has, during recent years, submitted himself to public demonstrations of cardiac catheterization on several occasions. But although this certainly establishes beyond question the professor's good faith, it does not prove that such a procedure is anything but uncomfortable or that it is entirely free from risk. Many men's professions and work involve them in discomfort and in some risk peculiar to that profession or work. They do not, however, expect the general public to undergo the same discomfort or run the same risk.

On the question of how far self-experimentation does or does not justify the repetition of the same experiments on others, it should be borne in mind that when the subject of an experiment is the experimenter himself then those who are conducting the procedure, who will be his colleagues and very likely also his subordinates, are likely to exercise particular care. So that although the element of risk may appear the same when the identical experiment is performed on others, yet it may actually be greater. If a mistake is made, and the doctor in charge is himself the subject, then there can be no concealing the fact. But if the subject is a patient and the same thing happens, then the fact that the complication which arose was someone's fault can be totally dissimulated. The legacy of a mistake in the procedure can then be represented to the sufferer as a symptom of his disease.

7. EXPERIMENTS ON NON-PATIENT VOLUNTEERS

There is certainly least objection to the use of medical students, young doctors, nurses and laboratory technicians, all of whom often volunteer to be the subjects of experiments. By the nature of their occupation these people are likely to have a reasonable and sometimes a complete understanding of what is being asked of them and of its possible consequences. But even here certain safeguards are necessary.

The fact that the subject of an experiment is a medical man does not obviate the necessity for any of the proper precautions and conditions.

Professor Mackintosh of the London School of Hygiene wrote to Dr. Beecher (the author of *Experimentation in Man*):

> On the difficult question of laboratory personnel we had certain decisions to make in the London School of Hygiene. In the study of malarial parasites in the human liver we had offers from a skilled technician to submit himself to infection and then to have a small liver section taken. In this case the technician was a senior man who was fully aware of the risks involved. His offer was gratefully accepted, but at the same time a regulation was passed that in future no human experiments should be allowed without a full report being made in advance to the School Council (which is the professional body) and to the Board of Management, which has a considerable representation of scientists and also lay members.

One danger with volunteers drawn from among students, young doctors and hospital personnel is that of a degree of coercion being exerted by the experimenter on the prospective volunteer, who is often in some way dependent on him. The person being invited to volunteer may, for instance, be a pupil of the professor of medicine who wants to go ahead with a particular investigation. Consequently he may feel either that he will reduce himself in his professor's eyes if he refuses, although he might refuse if it were not for this. Or he may feel that he can gain favour by coming forward promptly. These considerations, though often concealed, are not for that reason any the less real. They are clearly recognized by the recent recommendation of the World Medical Association which states:

> No doctor should lightly experiment on human beings when the subject of the experiment is in a dependent relation to the investigator, such as a medical student to his teacher or a technician in a laboratory to the head of his department.[1]

[1] *British Medical Journal*, 1962, **2**, 119.

What is Being Done

This same viewpoint had been previously even better stated by Professor Beecher,[1]

> Laboratory personel and medical students are often considered legitimate game for the eager investigator and certainly tradition has accepted their use. In my opinion there is reason why such groups are usually not a good choice. In a sense they are captive groups, not so seriously as prisoners of war, perhaps, but nonetheless available for certain kinds of subtle coercion. A volunteer should be just that, not one who may be subject to fear of the consequences if he does not co-operate. The more domineering the investigator, and thus the more valid the point made, the more likely is this possibility to be disclaimed. Denied or not, the situation does exist, and it is better to avoid it.

One safeguard which I think should always be strictly observed is that when an investigator asks students, technicians and similarly placed persons to volunteer he should always do so to the whole group and never to individuals separately. If a student is approached individually by his professor he may find it very embarrassing to refuse, although he does not freely wish to volunteer and has a perfect right not to. Pressures can also be exerted between equals and an otherwise unwilling subject may feel that he 'has to volunteer'. A case in point is that of one of my postgraduate students who was inveigled against his own better judgment into an experiment where the subjects were asked to take a radioactive strontium compound. Two other members of the same unit had already agreed to the procedure, and when he was approached as a third prospective subject he found it difficult to be the odd man out. Nevertheless his anxiety about the possible ill effects of the radioactive strontium on his bone marrow persisted and was not removed by reassurance from the experimenter.

I also think that where students or nurses under twenty-one are concerned, written consent from their parents should always be obtained.

The non-patient, like the patient invited to undergo an experiment, should always be fully informed of the risks involved;

[1] Professor H. K. Beecher, Professor of Anaesthesia, Harvard Medical School, Boston, Mass., *Experimentation in Man* (Springfield: Charles Thomas, 1959).

and it is the responsibility of the doctor in charge of the experiment, not of the volunteer submitting himself to it, to make sure that this is the case. In spite of the fact that the volunteer because he is healthy is often in a better position to assess the risks he is taking than a patient, there is strong suspicion that he does not always do so, and also that the experimenters are not always entirely candid about these risks.

In the following experiment on volunteers 'healthy male and female subjects of college age or younger', the aim was to see whether glandular fever could be transmitted.[1] Three possible methods of the transmission of this disease were tried out.

1. Throat washings from patients with glandular fever were sprayed into the nose and throat of the volunteer.
2. Blood from the same patients was injected (usually into the muscles) of the volunteers.
3. Preparations from the stools of the patients with glandular fever were introduced into the volunteers' stomachs via a tube.

Four of the subjects developed symptoms suggestive of a mild infection, but none definitely contracted the disease, which was an undesired result. This report makes no mention of parental consent and it is difficult to believe that the risks involved or the source of some of the material was fully explained. Glandular fever can have unpleasant complications, including meningitis.

Just as patients who are the subjects of experiments are often not fully informed of the extent of the proposed experiment, so the information given to non-patient volunteers is sometimes similarly incomplete. An example of this is the performance of kidney function tests, which necessitate intravenous infusions. In several cases known to me personally, and in others discussed in medical literature, the subject who has volunteered for this particular procedure – which he or she has clearly understood – has had a catheter passed into his or her bladder. This has come as a complete surprise to the volunteers, who had been led to expect only the intravenous infusion. A volunteer for one thing not infrequently finds that he has 'volunteered' for something else as well.

[1] A. S. Evans, of Yale University Medical School, *Journal of Clinical Investigation*, 1950, **29**, 508.

What is Being Done

The following are three examples of experiments undertaken on non-patient volunteers where, although they may have understood what was going to take place, the severity of the experience, or the risk attached, or both, were such that one feels that either the volunteering was done under pressure or the volunteers were very foolhardy.

The first is an experiment reported by Dr. Warren and others of Emery University, Atlanta, in 1945.[1] Twelve subjects who were doctors, students or paid volunteers underwent the following. A catheter was passed via an arm vein into the heart. A large needle was inserted into and kept in a femoral artery. A face mask with nose clip was fitted. When the heart output had been measured, between one and two pints of blood were taken from each subject and then two tourniquets were applied, one to each thigh, so as substantially to reduce the return of blood to the heart. By these means a condition equal to shock was produced in each subject.

Three of the subjects had 'acute circulatory collapse'. One subject underwent the experiment on three different occasions and it is reported that after the third 'he became ashen, began to sweat and complained of nausea'. He was then given an intravenous infusion of a pint of gelatin and, as a result of this, developed an extensive itchy rash. It is recorded that in five of the subjects the procedure caused a hyperactive circulation due to anxiety and that when the tourniquets were applied these subjects became pale and began to sweat profusely. One subject had a profound fall of blood pressure and complained that his hands and feet had become numb.

The subjects of the second experiment were a group of undergraduates who were first made to drink a large volume of water. They then had renal function tests done on them which included not only intravenous infusions but also bladder catheterization. 'The subjects were then placed on a tilt table . . . When the intended degree of circulatory collapse was reached, the subject was then returned to the horizontal' and the renal function tests repeated. The effects of the circulatory collapse which had been purposely produced was to seriously impair renal function for about ninety minutes. One student actually

[1] Warren, Brannon, E. A. Stead and A. J. Merrill, of Emery University Medical School, Atlanta, *Journal of Clinical Investigation*, 1945, **24**, 337.

84

developed anuria (acute kidney failure with no urine produced). Fortunately, he made an apparently complete recovery.[1]

The same doctors then repeated the same experiment on another group of students, but with the addition that when circulatory collapse had been produced in them a pint of blood was removed from each subject (which enhanced the collapse) and this blood was then transfused into the first group of students to see if it had any anti-diuretic properties.

The third experiment was the injection of adrenaline into a main artery of three volunteer students and into a main vein of three others. This procedure is not free from risk and many who have volunteered for such a procedure have personally informed me how unpleasant it was and how ill it made them feel. Although fatalities from intravenous adrenaline injections are comparatively rare, I myself have twice seen death result from precisely this. The risk from *intra-arterial* injections of adrenaline is greater. My particular purpose in quoting this experiment, however, is to show a special feature. It should be borne in mind that the subjects of the experiment, being medical students, would know something of the possible risks attaching to adrenaline. 'Emotional stress', says the report, 'was produced by leading the subject to believe that a wrong dose had been infused and that he was in considerable peril.' After allowing the subjects to endure the state of mind produced by this news for up to ten minutes, 'they were reassured'.[2]

This experiment highlights in vivid form the question: Can a person be a genuine volunteer to an experiment the exact nature of which is purposely kept from him?

The following excerpt from 'Pertinax' in the *British Medical Journal* cites an interesting case of the abuse of their position by research workers toward those in a dependent relation to them.[3]

Harvard University have dismissed two research workers for, according to *The Times*, 'involving a student in an experiment with psilocybin, a drug causing hallucinations and derived from mushrooms'. I feel sorry for these men, because they

[1] Brun, Knudson and Raaschou, of Copenhagen, *Journal of Clinical Investigation*, 1946, **25**, 48.
[2] W. E. Glover, Greenfield and R. G. Shanks, of Queen's University, Belfast. *Journal of Physiology*, 1962, **164**, 422.
[3] *British Medical Journal*, 1963, **1**, 1603.

were no doubt hot in the pursuit of truth – but apparently at the expense of someone in a dependent relationship to them. The W.M.A.'s provisional code of ethics specifically mentions the dangers of experimenting on those in a dependent relationship such as a student to his teacher and a laboratory attendant to his chief. It is important, I am convinced, to make such a code as detailed as possible, because the enthusiastic research worker will, without this check, persuade all and sundry with subtle casuistry that his actions are correct and essential. The great ploy is to say, 'It would have been unethical not to have done this experiment which is unethical.'

The following account was given by a postgraduate student of mine who witnessed in America a highly complex type of cardiac catheterization. The subject was a hard-up student who was paid for volunteering and had volunteered and been paid for similar experiments previously. During the present experiment the young man developed profound shock and collapse, followed by stoppage of the heart. He was successfully brought back to life, having, in fact, for a few moments been virtually dead. The experimenter then *continued with the experiment as though nothing had happened.* The experimenter's true attitude to his subject seems to have been expressed in the remark he made to those present at this performance: 'He must be a fool to repeatedly come back to us.'

The above case, like a number of those which I have deliberately cited in this book, is an extreme one. That does not, I am afraid, mean that it is unique in its offence against common morality. What it shows – and what I am trying to show – is the way in which standards of medical behaviour may deteriorate when they are allowed to. 'He must be a fool' probably originated from 'Well, why not?'

8. EXPERIMENTS ON PATIENTS AWAITING OPERATIONS AND AS EXTENSIONS OF OPERATIONS

Sometimes experiments are carried out on patients just before an operation or as an extension to an operation which is already being undertaken. The experimental procedure may be done shortly before the operation, say, the day before, and the patient may or may not be anaesthetized for the experiment. Or the experiment may be joined to the operation itself. The patient knows he is to undergo an operation, to which he has agreed, and it is natural for him to accept whatever is done to him as being connected with that operation. He thus may become an unsuspecting subject and a standing temptation to the experimenter.

Some surgeons wished to investigate the effect of general anaesthetics on liver blood flow.[1] As subjects for their study they chose eighteen patients, including a man of seventy, who were due to undergo major abdominal surgery. No further details of these patients are given in the report except that none of them had any disease of either heart or liver, the two types of disease to which information derived from this experiment might be relevant.

Before their operation these patients were submitted to hepatic vein catheterization (via the heart). This was done before the anaesthetic had been administered. The procedure necessitated the intravenous infusion of a dye and this part of the experiment must have occupied about an hour. The procedure was then repeated after the patients had received their general anaesthetics, but before surgery had been started.

The time that these patients spent under anaesthetic was therefore increased by about an hour. This cannot possibly be viewed as being in the interests of the patients, especially in the case of the man of seventy.

The following experiment is one of which I have read the published account several times with increasing amazement.[2] The subjects were eighteen patients described as undergoing either 'injection type lobotomy' (which is otherwise known as leucotomy and is a purposeful destruction of part of the white matter of the brain in an attempt to relieve mental symptoms); or 'cervico-thoracic sympathectomy' (a cutting of the sympathetic nerve in the neck and chest to relieve a variety of symptoms, including intractable pain); 'or other head and neck operations' not specified. None of the patients had any heart disease or any neurological disease other than mental. That is to say, none of them was suffering from a condition which the

---

[1] Shackman, Graber and Melrose, of Hammersmith Hospital, London, *Clinical Science*, 1953, **12**, 307.

[2] T. J. Bridges, Klemp Clark and Yahr, of Presbyterian and Frances Delafield Hospitals, New York, *Journal of Clinical Investigation*, 1958, **37**, 763.

results of the experiment were aimed at illuminating. The purpose of the experiment was, in fact, to record the effects of various procedures on brain circulation. The experiment was carried out prior to operation.

First, a small hole (known as a trephine) was made in the temporal region of the skull under local anaesthetic – presumably after the head had been partly or wholly shaved – and the membrane covering the brain was 'widely opened'. Next, a 'trephine button' was inserted into the skull through the trephine hole. From this 'button', tubes led to instruments which recorded cerebral circulation. This recording was done to show the effects of various procedures, namely, compression of the main veins of the neck; inhalation of a toxic gas (carbon dioxide); voluntary holding the breath for a considerable period; the intravenous injection of various substances, including nicotinic acid and also half a pint of ten per cent solution of alcohol. (This last I would consider in itself a dangerous procedure.)

This, however, was not all. The experimenters record that 'Apprehension was produced by threatening the patients with immersion of the left leg in iced water'. In some patients the experimenters recorded the effects on brain circulation of 'cutaneous pain'. (Two of the patients had abdominal cancer.) The experimenters comment, 'The trephine button may be left *in situ* (in place) indefinitely, avoiding the need to perform further surgery to remove the button.' And they add, 'It is possible to take records for up to twenty-three days.'

At the same hospital, in 1951, another experiment took place on thirty-four patients who were undergoing major surgery.[1] The aim of the experiment was to determine renal and hepatic blood flow during the administration of the anaesthetic, during the operation and immediately after. None of the patients, incidentally, had any liver, renal or cardiac disease.

A catheter was passed into the bladder of each patient and was repeatedly washed out during the experiment. An intravenous infusion was given and various samples of blood and urine were taken in order to estimate renal circulation. This procedure occupied about an hour. A catheter was then passed, via

[1] D. V. Habif, Papper, H. F. Fitzpatrick, P. Lowrance, Mc. C. Smythe and S. E. Bradley, of The Presbyterian Hospital, New York, *Surgery*, 1951, **30**, 241.

the arm, and through the heart into a vein in the liver. A dye was then infused intravenously. All this was done before giving the anaesthetic, which was then administered and the operation, for which these patients were in hospital in the first place, was begun. During the operation itself further blood samples were taken in order to remeasure renal and liver circulation. In the case of eleven patients similar studies were also continued from one to three hours after their operations.

Lung function tests on patients being operated on, after the anaesthetic had been given and before the actual operation was started, have also been reported.[1] The procedure involved the passage of a tube with a balloon at the end into the patient's gullet. Forty-four subjects were used of whom fourteen were studied before and then again during anaesthesia. None of the patients had a lung disease. The experimenters admit that these tests necessitated the giving of additional anaesthetic and additional muscle-relaxing drugs, but that 'No ill effects were noted in any case.'

Another experimental investigation done prior to operation was described as 'an incidental procedure during various surgical operations requiring laparotomy' (opening the abdomen). Whilst the patients were under the anaesthetic a catheter was passed into the portal vein which goes to the liver, and a contrast medium was injected through this and serial X-rays taken, so that the liver circulation could be studied. No details about the patients are given, not even the numbers involved, except that none had liver disease.[2]

A similar experiment to outline the liver veins was done on a group of twenty-one patients, 'during the course of exploratory laparotomy (opening the abdomen) or a definitive operation directed towards cure'. But the actual method was different because the contrast medium (40 c.c. of 35% diodrast) was injected directly into the exposed superior mesenteric vein which is a main vein of the colon and drains into the portal vein of the liver.[3]

[1] J. Butler and B. H. Smith, of Queen Elizabeth Hospital, Birmingham, England, *Clinical Science*, 1957, **16**, 125.

[2] G. E. Moore and Bridenbaugh, of University of Minnesota Hospital, Minneapolis, *Radiology*, 1951, **57**, 685.

[3] C. G. Child, Ward D. O'Sullivan, Mary Ann Payne and R. D. McClure, of New York Hospital-Cornell Medical Center, *Radiology*, 1951, **57**, 691.

What is Being Done

In 1958 the development of a new technique for measuring heart output was described.[1] This involved cardiac catheterization, the infusion intravenously of a solution containing a special radioactive substance, a wide-bore needle kept in a main artery and the application to the subject of a face mask and nose clip. The technique was first tried out on four anaesthetized dogs and then (the comparison of numbers is important) on eighty-six unanaesthetized adults. About these eighty-six patients no details are given except that none of them had cardiac failure or leaking valves. No statement is made regarding the patients' ages nor whether they had had or were awaiting operations.

All of this may be beyond suspicion, but there is always an inherent danger when a surgeon uses his patients, who have presumably been admitted to hospital to undergo operations, to develop techniques which are usually considered the province of the experimental physician.

A group of doctors wished to investigate the effect of various types of breathing on liver circulation.[2] The subjects chosen were nineteen patients who were undergoing minor surgery and none of whom had any heart, kidney or liver disease. These patients were first subjected to hepatic vein catheterization with the injection of a dye and also a radioactive compound into the catheter and various estimations were made prior to the actual operations.

Another experiment on twenty-two patients was to measure the amounts of circulating adrenaline under various specific conditions. Their ages ranged from fourteen to fifty-four, and they were either 'normal' patients or had small lung lesions.[3] Three other patients were also used on whom the experiment was conducted at the time when they were operated on for tumours of the chest.

The procedure was as follows. A catheter was passed into the right side of the heart, a wide-bore needle was inserted into the main arm artery and a tightly fitting face mask was applied. A dye was then injected directly into the pulmonary artery. Dur-

[1] Shackman, of Hammersmith Hospital, London, *Clinical Science*, 1958, **17**, 317.
[2] R. M. Epstein, H. O. Wheeler, M. J. Frumin, D. V. Habif, E. M. Papper and S. E. Bradley, of Presbyterian Hospital, New York, *Journal of Clinical Investigation*, 1961, **40**, 592.
[3] Goldring, Turino, G. Cohen, Jameson, G. B. Bass and A. P. Fishman, of Presbyterian Hospital, New York, *Journal of Clinical Investigation*, 1962, **41**, 1211.

ing the procedure 'brachial artery blood was withdrawn at a constant rate'. The three subjects who were studied at the time of their chest operations had needles inserted directly into their pulmonary artery and left atrial chamber of the heart and pressures recorded prior to and during a single rapid injection of adrenaline into the pulmonary artery. Otherwise the experiment consisted in measuring lung and heart function during four separate periods: (1) a control period immediately after the catheter had been inserted; this period lasted from ten to fifteen minutes; (2) a period of sixteen minutes during which the subject's respiration was markedly depressed by the inhalation of a special gas mixture; (3) a period lasting about an hour during which the patient received an intravenous infusion of noradrenaline; (4) a final period during which respiration was again depressed by the same technique while the noradrenaline infusion was still running. The authors explain that the patients were allowed to rest for fifteen to thirty minutes between each period. No doubt the three patients who were about to undergo surgery for tumours of the chest had given their permission for that operation. Had they also agreed to this lengthy, exhausing and unpleasant preliminary? Or did they imagine it was part of their necessary treatment?

A very important report of an experiment on children was published in 1964. The report is entitled 'Effects of thymectomy on skin graft survival'. Thymectomy is the removal of the whole or a part of a small gland called the thymus which is situated behind the breast-bone; it is present at birth, but gradually shrinks, and until recently was regarded as vestigial and without function. Recently, however, the thymus has been shown to have an important bearing on the development of immunity. This, in its turn, may be a crucial matter: whether or not any tissue transplanted from one person to another survives, as this also involves the problem of immunity response.[1]

In order to further investigate this association of the thymus, immunity and tissue transplantations, the following experiment was done. Eighteen patients, whose ages ranged from three and a half months to eighteen years, all of whom had congenital

[1] Zollinger, Linden, Filler, Corsor and R. E. Wilson, of Children's Hospital Medical Center and Peter Bent Brigham Hospital, Boston, *New England Journal of Medicine*, 1964, **270**, 707.

heart lesions, were admitted for surgery. We are informed that they were, 'selected randomly'. Immediately after the heart operation, eleven of them had a complete and seven a partial removal of their thymus. Skin grafts from other patients were then sutured into the wounds and their survival noted.

This report evoked a protest from Dr. B. H. Waksman, who asserted that in his view the experiment was ill considered and possibly dangerous, and should not have been even contemplated.[1]

He wrote,

> The thymus has a key role in development and maintenance of immunity . . . One may well question the value and propriety of studies like that of Zollinger in which total thymectomy is carried out as a purely experimental measure in subjects not having a disease to which this procedure is relevant . . .One may also ask if the long term hazards, unknown at present, were duly noted and called to the subjects' attention.

A report worthy of our notice was published in 1963. A forty-year-old married man presented himself in March 1962 for operation on a hernia. The previous year, at the same hospital, he had been found to be a diabetic and was put on insulin. The account of this patient contains the following statements:

> At the time of the investigation into the diabetes he was recognized as having a genital deformity about which he was so sensitive that he failed to keep an appointment at which it was hoped to investigate this aspect of his case.
> For this reason he was not questioned about his marital relationship at the time of admission for the hernia operation. Neither he nor his wife volunteered any further information about the matter, and it was not thought to be in his interests to worry him further. It was decided to examine his genitalia very closely under anaesthesia at the time of the hernia operation.
> The hernia sac was explored and opened. Within it the found recognizable structures were a rudimentary uterus and one Fallopian tube. (Proving 'he' was really a woman.) . . .

[1] B. H. Waksman, *New England Journal Medicine*, 1964, **270**, 1018.

92

The abdomen was then opened and the pelvis inspected. No other genital organs could be found.

We do not propose to discuss in any details the management of hermaphroditism. This patient was a 40 year old and married man who wanted treatment for his hernia. It is clear that he had nothing to gain, and perhaps much to lose, by our paying more than a passing attention to this aspect of his case.[1]

The surgeon also passed a cystoscope, an instrument with a light at its end, for examination of the interior of the bladder. This is not a normal part of any hernia operation but was done to see whether or not the bladder was of a female type.

This report concludes:

We wish to thank Mr. Masina, under whose care the patient was admitted and who performed the operation, for permission to study and report this case.

A doctor wrote to the medical journal which printed this report and asked the following pertinent questions.

But for the sake of science, would the cystoscopy and laparotomy (opening of the abdomen) have been performed upon an important influential patient, or upon a personal friend, or upon a close relation? And where does the family doctor stand?[2]

No replies to these questions were ever published.

In order to study the effects of anaesthetics on the liver, two doctors did liver punctures on seventy patients whilst they were undergoing major upper abdominal surgery.[3]

9. THE DANGERS OF EXPOSURE TO RADIATION

Risks of radiation exposure can be incurred by patients being subjected either to X-rays or radioactive isotopes. X-rays are used for diagnostic investigations, for research techniques, and

[1] Dewhurst, Warrack and M. D. Casey, of City General Hospital, Sheffield, *British Medical Journal*, 1963, **2,** 221.
[2] O. L. S. Scott, *British Medical Journal*, 1963, **2,** 621.
[3] K. S. Kemley and G. C. Corssen, of University of Michigan, Ann Arbor, *Therapeutic Agents and the Liver* (Blackwell, 1965) (edited by McIntyre and S. Sherlock).

for treatment. I do not intend to discuss the dangers of X-rays used in treatment, especially of cancer. The outlook almost always warrants the risks involved.

The effects of radiation depend on the dosage, the duration and frequency of exposure, and the tissue exposed. But in any case the effects are somatic (direct effects on the person's own body) and/or genetic (not on the individual exposed but on his or her future children).

The commonest and most important somatic radiation damage is to the bone marrow, as a result of which the proper development of the red and the white blood cells, and also the platelets (which are necessary for proper blood clotting), are all severely depressed or even abolished altogether, with serious or even fatal consequences.

Other somatic effects are seen in reduced fertility due to exposure of the gonads (ovaries or testes), increased incidence of all types of tumours, especially leukaemia, and reduction in the lifespan.

The genetic effects, which are not seen in the individual exposed, but may be handed on as damage to subsequent generations, may show themselves at birth in gross deformations of the limbs, brain or other internal organs, or as less definite damage later in life, such as diabetes or impaired mental ability.

Both somatic and genetic effects may occur when the foetus (the baby in the womb) is exposed to radiation, and for some of the long-term effects the foetus may be several times more sensitive than the mother. Such exposure may occur inadvertently in the earliest stages of pregnancy, when neither the radiographer nor the patient may be aware of it. It is for this reason that the International Committee on Radiological Protection recommend that where possible a woman of child-bearing age should only be X-rayed in the first ten days after a period, when she is extremely unlikely to be pregnant.

A more controversial problem is the relationship of exposure to X-rays and the subsequent development of leukaemia. A recent leading article in the *British Medical Journal*[1] referred to an alarming increase of about 50% in the number of deaths from leukaemia during the period 1945 to 1961, and mentioned

[1] *British Medical Journal*, 1964, **1**, 384.

the possibility of the increased use of X-rays as a causative factor. The statistical evidence of this marked increase in leukaemia incidence has not been seriously disputed, but the trend is world-wide. It has taken place also in those countries where there has not been much increase in the use of X-rays, and, therefore, this can be only one possible factor responsible for the increased leukaemia frequency.

A recent report from the British Medical Research Council expresses this authoritative opinion:

> It is now generally accepted, however, that in assessing the possible risks from low dose exposures, for which the effect can only be guessed from the information of leukaemia and cancer incidence following high dose exposures, a finite risk per unit dose, must be accepted. This is estimated as 20–40 extra cases of fatal cancer per million population per unit dose (rad). This is over and above the present level of 2200 cases per million persons per year. Because of lack of data these may be overestimates of risk, but give a yardstick for assessment of relative risk and advantage from radiation exposure.[1]

All X-ray procedures, whatever their nature, undoubtedly carry some risk. With a simple procedure such as ordinary X-ray of chest or of a bone, this risk is so slight as to be almost non-existent, but with more complicated procedures, requiring more frequent and/or prolonged exposures, the risk is markedly increased. The good prudent doctor must always balance those possible risks against the possible diagnostic value of the investigation. Unfortunately there is a rapidly growing and ever-increasing tendency both in America and Great Britain for a needless proliferation of X-ray examinations and overinquisitive unnecessary radiology is far too common. Far too few clinicians ask themselves, 'Is the proposed X-ray investigation really necessary?' and, if not, would it not be better in the patient's own interests (time and expense as well as health) not to order the suggested X-rays?

The recent report of the Adrian Committee[2] among its

[1] *Medical Research Council Report from Committee on Protection against Ionizing Radiations* (H.M.S.O., London, 1966).
[2] *Radiological Hazards to Patients* (Second Report of the Committee, H.M.S.O., 1960).

recommendations states that:

(*a*) There should be clear-cut clinical indications before any X-ray examination is undertaken, and it should be ascertained whether there has been any previous radiological examination which would make further examination unnecessary. For this purpose the case sheet should have a section labelled 'previous X-rays'.

(*c*) All requests for examinations should state precisely the clinical indications and the information required.

(*d*) There should be consultation between clinician and radiologist before extensive or repeated radiological examinations of young individuals are undertaken. It must be realized that radiological exposure is just as much the responsibility of the clinician as of the radiologist.

(*f*) Special precautions should be adopted in the radiography of pregnant women. Only essential examinations should be carried out during pregnancy and particular care should be taken to avoid irradiation of the foetus whenever possible. In all women of child-bearing age the clinician requesting the examination should never overlook the possibility of early pregnancy.

Mention must be made of special procedures done under 'X-ray control'. For example, when a catheter is passed along a vein or artery into a heart chamber or other organ, the passage of the catheter, which is especially made opaque to X-rays, is guided behind an X-ray screen on which the physician can see the image of the catheter and the organ to be catheterized. The time taken to pass the catheter will depend on the inherent difficulties of the technique used and the skill of the doctor, but may take as long as an hour or even more, the patient being exposed to X-rays all the time. When the catheter is finally positioned a contrast medium is usually injected through it and serial X-rays (perhaps four, perhaps over twenty) are taken, thus exposing the patient to still more radiation.

An indication of the actual dose of radiation received in terms of benefit to the patient from the examination, can be seen by comparison with chest X-rays, where the advantages of early diagnosis of infectious diseases, such as T.B., are obvious to both the individual and the community.

From a straight chest X-ray, the skin will receive about 0.2

rad, and the bone marrow, important from the leukaemia risk, 0.01 rad. For cardiac catheterization, however, the skin dose can be about 7 rad, and the bone marrow dose about 1 rad, that is 100 times greater than for a chest X-ray. These are average figures and can be significantly greater or smaller depending on the skill of the operators and the length of time the procedure takes.

When such complex radiological procedures are used for research purposes, that is, not directly for the patient's own benefit, it behoves the doctor to consider even more carefully, and with genuine searching of his conscience, the advisability of exposing patients, who are often in complete ignorance that there is any risk whatsoever, to prolonged radiation. It is my considered opinion after repeated inquiries that too many research doctors completely ignore the possibilities of radiological hazards, so keen are they to achieve their research results. A great difficulty is that many such investigations are performed in the ill-defined territory where genuinely diagnostic investigations and pure research mingle. The unscrupulous investigators take advantage of this lack of clear demarcation, claiming their investigations to be genuine and necessary diagnostic procedures.

It is true that during the last few years closed-circuit television monitors and image intensifiers have been two important advances reducing the hazards of X-rays. But these are both very expensive pieces of equipment possessed by very few hospitals, and their cost for widespread use would be prohibitive.

A point often overlooked is that many experimental physicians using complex radiological techniques are rarely themselves qualified radiologists and yet take charge of the X-ray apparatus during the experiment. Some have been supplied with their own X-ray equipment so that they can act independent of a radiologist. Such doctors, sometimes from ignorance, are less likely to avoid the possible dangers of X-rays than the trained radiologist.

At the end of 1964 a code of practice was published by Her Majesty's Stationery Office[1] for the protection of persons exposed to ionizing radiation in research and teaching.

[1] *Code of Practice for the Protection of Persons Exposed to Ionizing Radiations in Research and Teaching* (H.M.S.O., 1964).

2.4.1. It must be impressed on every individual working with ionizing radiations or radioactive substances that he has a duty to protect both himself and others from any hazard arising from his work and that he must not expose himself or others to ionizing radiations to a greater extent than is reasonably necessary for the purposes of work.

This is reinforced in the Code for Medical and Dental Practice drawn up by another Panel of the Radioactive Substances Advisory Committee, in which a line of responsibility is laid down for the use of radiation either in therapy or diagnosis.

Recently these Codes came into force, but obviously there are still administrative difficulties due to lack of appropriate staff and funds, which lead to inevitable loopholes.

A recent report from the United Nations Organization[1] contains the following conclusions:

50. At present even the wide use of radiation in medical diagnosis and treatment in countries with extensive medical facilities does not usually involve more than about a 50 per cent increase in the genetically significant exposure to radiation of their populations, and there is evidence that simple and inexpensive modifications of techniques could reduce the figure considerably without loss of medically important information. 52. The Committee therefore emphasizes the need that all forms of unnecessary radiation exposure should be minimized or avoided entirely, particularly when the exposure of large populations is entailed; and that every procedure involving the peaceful uses of ionizing radiation should be subject to appropriate immediate and continuing scrutiny in order to ensure that the resulting exposure is kept to the minimum practicable level and that this level is consistent with the necessity or the value of the procedure.

It is extremely easy to accept these average levels on the basis, but it must also be remembered that these will not include individual cases of overexposure or abuses of radiation in medical research, as these were not used for routine monitoring of patient dose in these international surveys.

Radioactive isotopes are being used more and more in medicine both for purely experimental purposes and for diag-

[1] *UNSCEAR* Supplement 16 (A/5216) (U.N., New York, 1962).

nosis. The dangers of these isotopes are the effects on the special sites of their accumulation and action, for example, radioactive iodine on the thyroid and radioactive strontium on bones. In large doses they produce irreversible destruction of the particular organ or tissue. In moderate doses they may initiate malignant processes.

In Great Britain, rightly and fortunately, all radioactive isotopes are under the control of the Medical Research Council and nobody can obtain supplies without agreement from that organization and scrutiny of the purpose for which they are asked. Moreover, the Medical Research Council insists that any experimental use must be designed by a competent approved physicist or radiologist. In the U.S.A. no such strict control is generally applied. This is a serious legislative omission demanding urgent action. Some quotations should indicate this.

Radioactive iodine is commonly used for the investigation of thyroid function. A recent American article[1] which discusses the dangers of radiation points out that many clinicians have been chary of giving radioactive iodine to children because of the undoubted risk of its producing cancer in the thyroid gland. Yet one of the authors of this same warning, together with some other colleagues, described the intravenous administration for purely experimental purposes of radioactive iodine to forty-six healthy newborn infants, in order to study thyroid function in the newborn. No other details about these infants are given.[2]

Incidentally, in the same medical journal, the dangers of repeated X-rays taken of children with heart disease and the performance on them of techniques which require X-ray control are fully discussed. The authors express the opinion.[3]

> These children may be subjected to multiple chest X-rays, repeated fluoscopies, prolonged exposures during cardiac catheterization, and as many as 20 to 60 films at one or more angiocardiographic examinations.

The editorial comment in the same issue of that journal,

[1] A. Fisher and Panos, of Medical Center, Little Rock, Arkansas, *American Journal Diseases of Children*, 1962, **103**, 729.

[2] D. A. Fisher, Oddie and J. C. Burroughs, of Little Rock, Arkansas, *American Journal Diseases of Children*, 1962, **103**, 739.

[3] M. S. Spach and M. P. Capp, of Duke University School of Medicine, N.C., *American Journal Diseases of Children*, 1962, **103**, 750.

refers to all three of these articles and warns against the 'premature use of technological advances' and continues:

> So too for radioactive iodine and tests of its uptake. Most often
> it is given in good faith. Good faith no longer suffices. Just as
> a baby with pulmonary infiltration (shown on an X-ray) and
> a positive tuberculin test has tuberculosis and does not need
> lung biopsy to determine whether it is due to human or the
> bovine strain of tuberculosis, thyroid disease can be diagnosed
> and superbly managed without resource to radioactive iodine.
> The old shibboleth, 'It would be interesting' certainly is
> outdated if risk is involved, especially in children. Even in re-
> search centres potential risk is acceptable only after all other
> avenues have been explored.
> As we see it, the Russians with their 30 to 50 megaton display
> gave British infants (as estimated by radioactive iodine in milk,
> see *British Medical Journal*, 1961, **2,** 1275), perhaps as much as
> one eighth as much thyroid radiation as the small dose of
> radioactive iodine mentioned by Fisher as 'acceptable'.
> Whether this alarms you or tranquilizes you undoubtedly
> depends on your point of view.

The following experiment was done in order to determine
how rapidly and effectively newborn babies could dispose of
radioactive compounds.[1] To quote from the authors themselves:

> If following the injection of radioactive material to a mother,
> a large part of the dose were to cross the placenta (after-birth),
> we had to be assured that the newborn would dispose of the
> compound as rapidly as the normal adults do. Therefore in
> the first step in the present study, we measured the urinary
> excretion of radioactivity during the 48 hours following the
> administration of minimal dose to 2 newborns, 15 and 20 hours
> of age. Since the excretions were within normal limits it was
> considered safe to proceed with the injection of mothers shortly
> before delivery.

The research team thus first administered a radioactive compound to two babies less than a day old. When it was found
that, in these two cases, radioactivity was dispersed within
forty-eight hours, which is regarded as safe for adults, the

[1] Migeon, Bertrand and Patricia Wall, of Department of Pediatrics, Johns
Hopkins, Baltimore, *Journal Clinical Investigation*, 1957, **36,** 1350.

experimenters proceeded to inject the mothers shortly before delivery. The subjects now chosen to continue this experiment were nine women awaiting delivery by Caesarean section. These were given radioactive material by intravenous injection from twenty-four to forty-eight hours before their operations in three cases; and less than an hour and a quarter before their operation in the other six cases. The report states that samples of blood and urine were taken from both mothers and babies (presumably collected by bladder catheterization). What has to be justified is the use of newborn infants to test the possible toxic effects of radioactive compounds.

10. PATIENTS AS CONTROLS

In the present chapter I shall describe a number of experiments of which the main feature is the use of patients as controls. Where a patient is used as a control it means that he himself is free from the disease or condition which the experiment he undergoes is designed to investigate. As a result of experimenting on controls, the experimenter hopes to establish certain normal conditions and reactions which will provide a basis for comparison with the abnormal ones that may accompany the disease he is investigating.

For example, an investigator may wish to find out what changes occur in the blood pressures in the left chambers of the heart when a patient is suffering from a particular heart disease. Or he may wish to determine how the blood supply to the liver or to some other organ is affected by a disease of that organ. In order to do this he will need to establish, not only the particular pressures and supply in patients who are suffering from these diseases but also these values in people free from the diseases. To find out these 'normals' the investigator uses controls.

The control subject is nearly always a hospital patient, sick with, and being treated for, a disease of his own (which has no relation to the one being investigated). Such a subject may be submitted to more than one investigation (as a control in each case) simultaneously. For example, he may undergo catheterization of the liver via the heart – to obtain blood samples from the liver – and at the same time have a needle inserted into his spleen in order to measure blood pressures in that organ. And the whole of these joint procedures, which are certainly unpleasant even if they are not dangerous, may, and often does, take over three hours.

The use of hospital patients in this way raises once again the ethical problems involved in research. The obtaining of the free and informed consent of patients used as controls is even more important than it is with healthy people who may be used in the same way. To a person in good health the discomfort, which is often inseparable from an experiment, is far more easily borne than it is by someone already sick; while the hazards which are also often inseparable from an experiment – certainly from some – are likely to be less in someone in good health than they will be in someone who is sick. Moreover, there is a greater temptation to use a sick person in hospital as a control than to use a healthy one. To a healthy person an explanation of some kind and his consent are obviously essential. But a sick person in hospital could be submitted to an experiment without having it put clearly to him at all. He could simply be allowed to think that what he is undergoing is part of the investigations for which he entered hospital. And frequently this is exactly what does happen. Where patient controls are concerned, consent is frequently not asked for and the fact that what is being done is an experiment quite unrelated to the patient's own disease or condition is frequently not revealed to him at all.

No doubt in a number of instances the real nature of what is proposed and the possible hazards are explained to the patient, who is then invited to act as a control. But there are an enormous number of cases where such points are excluded from any explanation given to the patient and very many where no such explanation is offered at all.

I myself teach a large number of medical postgraduates who have, of course, completed their normal time in hospital as students. Their first-hand reports confirm only too well what I have seen myself. Adequate, let alone full, explanations are often not given to patients. Possible complications and real dangers are hardly ever hinted at. What commonly happens is that Dr. X tells his colleagues and junior staff that he wants so many patients for a control series. The junior doctors are then ordered to 'find' these control patients. Often the experimenters have never even talked to the patient prior to the experiment, let alone explained anything, let alone asked consent. In some hospitals even the house physicians may be unaware of what is happening to some of their patients and do not know why, for example, a certain patient is missing from his ward on a certain day.

What is specially deplorable is the attitude of some doctors who regard hospital patients as somehow part of their possessions, as material conveniently available for their personal use in the furtherance of science. This attitude is well described and criticized by Professor Ross Mitchell in an article in which he comments on the former use of orphans as research material.[1]

> After 1900 . . . references (in descriptions of medical experiments) to orphans and foundlings gradually diminish. Despite this reports seldom referred to the obtaining of permission except, curiously enough, from medical staff. Thus there were frequent acknowledgements in the early pediatric journals of the kindness of obstetric staff in giving permission for experiments on their cases – a possessiveness which still exists to some extent today amongst doctors, as though the undertaking of medical care somehow conferred ownership of the patient on the physician.

Finally, the use of control patients often means that such patients are kept in hospital longer than would otherwise have been necessary. And since, as I mentioned earlier, experiments in England are confined to what is known as the 'hospital class' and not carried out on private patients, it follows that the deprivation of a few more days' health and the consequent probable loss of income, because the person cannot get back to his job for that time, falls precisely on those who can afford it least.

In 1956 the following experiment was carried out.[2] Thirty patients, aged fourteen to sixty-seven, were selected as subjects for calcium metabolism studies because they had X-ray evidence, though often slight, of bone disease. To these patients the experiment could legitimately be regarded as relevant. Sixty-eight other patients, who were without any bone disease, were employed as controls.

[1] *British Medical Journal*, 1964, **1,** 721.
[2] Nordin and Russel Fraser, of Hammersmith Hospital, London, *Lancet*, 1956, **1,** 823.

What is Being Done

(The reader may be surprised at the size of the control group used in this experiment and in some others, and not without reason. For experimental teams, in order to obtain large numbers which will be 'statistically significant', seem to err on the side of excess in deciding how many subjects, and particularly how many control subjects, they really need.)

The sixty-eight patient controls who were used on the present occasion are described in the report as having been convalescent from 'acute illnesses, e.g. coronary thrombosis, acute nephritis, pneumonia, cerebral thrombosis, or had chronic diseases'.

All the subjects were put on a low calcium diet for three days and were then given an infusion of calcium over a four-hour period. Numerous blood samples were taken. On seven of these patients the experiment was done more than once. The report of this experiment did not mention whether the control patients or, indeed, the others, had given their consent and the question of whether in fact their consent had been sought was raised by Dr. Ryle in the same issue of the *Lancet*. He asked:

> Would it not be a good principle to state clearly in all accounts of experiments utilizing human controls that the human controls are volunteers and to record the means by which their co-operation was achieved?[1]

The experimenters replied:

> With all patients, agreement to the performance of the procedure was of course obtained. We had every reason to believe that the test was devoid of any risk.

The use of the word 'any' in this context is surely a gross exaggeration. Infusion of large amounts of fluid into patients with heart or kidney disease must always carry with it a risk which is well recognized by practising clinicians.

Similar calcium infusions were done at the same hospital by another team of research physicians on a group of twenty-five patients who had chronic jaundice. In one patient the jaundice was due to secondary cancer deposits in the liver and in five others it was due to cancer of the bile ducts, including a woman of seventy-seven. In addition to the prolonged procedure outlined in the previous experiment, the patients had a small

[1] *Lancet*, 1956, 2, 1012.

portion of their iliac (pelvic) bone removed for microscopic examination.[1]

A group of physicians set out to investigate 'the characteristics of peripheral transport of radioactive palmitic acid.'[2] To do so they injected the material intravenously into sixteen hospital patients 'who were all free from serious disease', except one. This last patient was speechless and paralysed due to a progressive nervous disease, and into him was injected, over a three-hour period, ten times the amount of the radioactive substance given to the other patients.

In 1949 there was carried out an extensive experiment on a large number of patients who included a control group numbering thirty-four.[3] The aim of the experiment was to study liver and muscle chemistry in diabetes and liver disease, the 'direct' subjects of the experiment being patients who were suffering from one or the other of these conditions. The procedure consisted in making an incision over both pectoral muscles of the chest and over the gastrocnemius muscles of the calves, through which small pieces of muscle were removed at frequent intervals. Chemical estimations of the pieces of muscle so removed were then made. At the same time most of the patients were submitted to liver puncture.

The report describes the thirty-four control patients as 'convalescing'. One of them, however, had cancer of the lung, one cancer of the colon, a third leukaemia and a fourth Paget's disease of the bone (a progressive and incurable condition). It is difficult to see how these four could have been 'convalescing'. It is stated that 'after a simple explanation the patients gave permission for the procedure'.

In the same issue of the journal the same doctors describe a further experiment, of a very similar nature, in which use was again made of 'convalescing controls'. This time the control group numbered nineteen, of whom six had already taken part in the experiment just described. The six subjected to both experiments included the patient with cancer of the colon.

[1] M. Atkinson, Nordin and Sherlock, of Hammersmith Hospital, London, *Quarterly Journal Medicine*, 1956, **25**, 299.
[2] S. J. Freidberg, R. F. Klein, Tront, Bogdonoff and Estes, of Duke University, Durham, N.C., *Journal Clinical Investigation*, 1960, **39**, 1511.
[3] Hilden, Sheila Sherlock and Veryan Walshe, of Hammersmith Hospital, London, *Clinical Science*, 1949, **7**, 287, 292.

Among the others were patients suffering from cancer of the lung, Parkinsonian paralysis, motor neurone disease (with paralysis of all limbs and tongue and throat muscles), arthritis (a patient aged seventy), psychoneurosis, and 'depressive psychosis'.

In this experiment the procedure was extended, and after the initial chemical estimations of liver and muscle samples had been made, the patients were given for a period of one hour an intravenous infusion containing adrenaline. The muscle biopsies and liver punctures were then repeated. At least five of the control group had liver punctures before and after the adrenaline infusions. Some patients also had a catheter kept in the bladder throughout the experiment, which lasted over three hours.

In 1958 some studies on sugar metabolism were undertaken. For the investigation twenty-seven 'mildly ill patients', most of whom had gastric disturbances were used, and, in addition, a control group of sixteen patients whom the report describes as 'normal', but about whom no further details are given. The procedure was as follows. A catheter was passed via an arm vein into and through the heart and so into the hepatic vein of the liver. A large-bore needle was inserted into the femoral artery. Through another needle, inserted into a femoral vein, a dye was injected. For the next hour the patients received an intravenous infusion of sodium octonate and samples of blood were taken from the hepatic vein, the femoral vein and the femoral artery, at five-minute intervals.[1]

The same experiment was later repeated on six patients described as 'neurotic', but in their case the procedure was extended. After the same process as the above, these six patients were given an injection of insulin (intravenously) so as to produce a 'brisk but brief hypoglycaemia' (lowering of the blood sugar). The whole experiment was then repeated on a still further group of seven 'neurotics', with the variation that these last subjects were given cortisone prior to being rendered hypoglycaemic.

Complex heart and lung tests on thirty-three patients who, according to the report, had no 'cardiac or pulmonary or other

[1] H. T. McPherson, Werk, J. D. Myers and Engel, of Duke University Medical School, *Journal Clinical Investigation*, 1958, **37**, 1379.

serious disease', and who may, therefore, be regarded as being purely controls, was reported in 1961.[1] First, a catheter was passed via an arm vein into the main chest vein, the superior vena cava, almost as far as the right atrial heart chamber. Face masks were then fitted together with nose clips so that samples of expired air could be obtained. A large needle was inserted into and kept in a main limb artery. A dye was then injected via the catheter. When the required estimations had been made, the patients, with catheter and face mask still in position, were made to exercise vigorously and the estimations were then repeated.

This completed the first stage of the experiment. For fourteen of the patients, however, a further stage followed immediately. This was the intravenous injection of a drug called lantoside C, which acts very powerfully on the heart. The cardiac output of these fourteen patients was then measured at 'frequent intervals' for up to two hours after giving the injection'. For thirteen other patients stage two of the experiment consisted in administering digitalis, which also has a powerful action on the heart, for seven days. At the end of that time the whole experiment, necessitating cardiac catheterization and lung function tests, was repeated.

In 1948 there was published an account of an investigation into the effects on renal function of giving a high spinal anaesthetic to fourteen patients with cardiac failure.[2] No reason other than the purely experimental one is given for submitting these patients to this procedure, and the subjects used must, therefore, be regarded as a control group. In view of their very sick condition it is difficult to justify the decision to use these subjects for such an unpleasant procedure. The gravity of the subjects' condition is emphasized by the fact that, in some cases, they were so short of breath that the lumbar punctures had to be done with the patient sitting up instead of in the more usual position of the patient lying flat. One patient was a girl of sixteen. The report states that in several instances the anaesthesia reached the first thoracic segment (i.e. high up on

[1] Rodman, Gorezyea and Pastor, of Veterans' Hospital, Philadelphia, *Annals of Internal Medicine*, 1961, **55**, 620.
[2] Mokotoff and George Ross, of Montefiore Hospital, New York City, *Journal Clinical Investigation*, 1948, **27**, 335.

the chest). In these cases, because of the paralysis of chest muscles so induced, oxygen had to be administered.

Had the consent of any of these patients been obtained? If so, were the dangers, including that of the temporary paralysis of chest muscles, mentioned to them? The authors of the report are silent on both of these points.

In 1950 an experiment of which the aim was to investigate sugar metabolism was done.[1] The procedure was, first, the passing of a catheter via an arm vein through the right side of the heart into the hepatic vein. Next a large-bore needle was inserted in the femoral artery; a dye was then infused via the catheter. Blood samples were then taken from the hepatic vein and femoral artery. When this had been done the patients were given intravenous injections of glucose and the performance was repeated.

The 'direct' subjects of this experiment were: eighteen patients with cirrhosis of the liver; ten with active thyrotoxicosis (a disease which produces marked nervousness); nine with diabetes; and eight with cardiac failure. A control group of thirty-eight patients was also used, these patients being described in the report as 'with no or insignificant disease' and about whom no further information is given. Of the total of eighty-five patients involved, only in the case of the eighteen with cirrhosis of the liver could this experiment be said to have any relevance. The authors record that 'the entire procedure was generally accomplished without significant discomfort'. It would be of interest to know precisely what is intended by 'generally' and by 'significant' in this context.

The following experiment is of interest.[2] Forty-nine patients were given potassium iodine for three days. They were then submitted to hepatic vein catheterization and at the same time a second catheter was passed into the femoral artery of the thigh.

When these catheters were in position the patients were given an intravenous infusion of a radioactive substance. Samples of blood were then taken from the hepatic vein, from the femoral

[1] J. D. Myers, of Duke University Medical School, *Journal of Clinical Investigation*, 1950, **29,** 1421.
[2] Shaldon, Chiandussi, Guevera, Caesar and Sheila Sherlock, of Royal Free Hospital, London, *Journal of Clinical Investigation*, 1961, **40,** 1346.

artery, and also from the vein of the forearm during a period of thirty minutes. In this time nine samples were taken from each of these three sites. In the case of some patients further samples were taken for up to an hour. In the case of one patient samples were taken four-hourly for twenty-four hours, the catheters presumably being left in position throughout the whole of that period, although the report is not entirely clear on that point.

The patients who underwent this experiment were thirty-two with cirrhosis of the liver, three with thrombosis of one of the main liver veins, but with otherwise normal livers, and a control group of fourteen patients. Of these fourteen controls, four had gastric ulcers; one had neurosis; one had sarcoidosis. No details were given of the other eight.[1] If the patients were genuine volunteers, I should like to have heard what explanation was given to them as to the nature of the proposed very complicated and hazardous experiment.

Investigation of abdominal blood flow by the technique of liver vein catheterization under X-ray control has been described.[2] This involved the infusion of a dye intravenously and the insertion of an indwelling needle into an arm vein. The subjects of this experiment were forty-nine patients who 'had no known hepatic dysfunction' and whose ages ranged from twenty to seventy-five.

A further experiment of which the purpose was to study the effects of intravenous adrenaline on liver blood flow was later reported.[3] Twenty-two patients were used about whom no details are given apart from the fact that they did not have liver disease. They may, therefore, be regarded as controls. These patients were put on a fast for twelve hours, after which a catheter was passed via the heart into the hepatic vein. A needle was inserted into an arm vein and after a dye had been infused through the catheter the adrenaline was injected into a

[1] All the patients with liver disease were, in addition, submitted to splenic venography (the insertion of a needle into the spleen and the injection of a contrast medium into it, followed by serial X-rays).

[2] Sheila Sherlock, Bearn, Barbara Billing (non-medical) and J. C. S. Paterson of Hammersmith Hospital, London, *Journal of Laboratory and Clinical Medicine*, 1950, 35, 923.

[3] Bearn, Barbara Billing and Sheila Sherlock, of Hammersmith Hospital, London, *Journal of Physiology*, 1951, 115, 430.

vein. Frequent samples were taken from the hepatic vein and from the arm vein. The experiment lasted over three hours.

In a further paper published in 1953 some doctors report a study on the effects of hexamethonium (a drug which causes a profound lowering of blood pressure) on abdominal circulation.[1] A group of seventeen patients was used for this purpose, about whom no details are given except their ages (one was seventy-one) and the fact that five had high blood pressure. None of them had liver disease. The hepatic vein was cathete-ized and a dye infused through this catheter. A second catheter was kept in the brachial artery for blood sampling. After pre-liminary measurements and blood samples from liver vein and arm artery were taken, the hexamethonium was injected intra-muscularly and further samples were taken. The fall of blood pressure produced was considerable. (The average fall was 32%, but in one patient it fell to 50% of normal.) Sudden falls of blood pressure, especially in elderly people, can have very serious consequences, causing clotting in brain or heart arteries. The duration of the experiment was three to four hours, except in the case of six of the patients, where it lasted beyond that period.

In 1953 an expert on liver diseases reported that in a two-year period she had done over two hundred hepatic vein catheterizations, but how many of these patients did not have liver disease and were controls is not stated. In the same paper is described an experiment of which the aim was to assess pressures in the portal vein (the main vein bringing blood to the liver from the abdominal viscera).[2] Eleven patients with cirrhosis of the liver were used and as a control series a group of twenty-eight patients who were without liver disease, which included four with cardiac failure. The report states that these twenty-two patients were those in whom 'cardiac catheteriza-tion for a necessary assessment of cardiovascular, metabolic or renal function was considered necessary'. In other words the use of the control group for this complex experiment was considered justified because the patients in question had already had

[1] T. B. Reynolds, A. Paton, M. Freeman, F. Howard and Sheila Sherlock, of Hammersmith Hospital, London, *Journal of Clinical Investigation*, 1953, **32**, 793.

[2] A. Paton, T. B. Reynolds and Sheila Sherlock, of Hammersmith Hospital, London, *Lancet*, 1953, **1**, 918.

cardiac catheterization done on them by someone else; that procedure having been completed, an investigation was made in the form of an extension of the original one. But what about consent? Consent to cardiac catheterization, presuming that this had been given, does not entitle a second investigator to perform *hepatic* catheterization. Moreover, I do not know any metabolic or renal disease in which cardiac catheterization can be legitimately considered a 'necessary assessment'.

In all of these patients the cardiac catheter was passed through the heart and then wedged ten centimetres beyond the mouth of the hepatic vein. We are informed that 'the whole procedure of hepatic vein catheterization rarely last longer than forty-five minutes'. But to gauge the complexity of the whole technique, it should be borne in mind that this comprises only the initial part of the procedure. Also, the timing referred to here applies to an expert. With the not-so-expert this time is likely to be considerably longer. Blood samples were taken at frequent and regular intervals for two hours after the completion of the catheterization.

A further quotation from this report is illuminating:

> In some patients submitted to operation the opportunity was taken to measure the pressure in the portal vein more directly. A polythene tube was inserted at operation into a tributary of the portal vein and tied in position. At the end of the operation it was brought out through a separate stab wound and stitched to the skin. Pressure measurements were made for the first few days after the operation.

Further studies of the effects of hexamethonium on liver circulation were published, but on this occasion the drug was injected during a state of hypoglycaemia induced by insulin.[1] The subjects in this case were twelve patients free from both liver disease and diabetes, whose ages ranged from twenty-seven to sixty-seven, but no details of their illnesses are given. 'They were studied during the course of catheterization for other conditions.' The procedure was taken over from the initial investigator and the catheter passed farther through the heart into the hepatic vein.

[1] Billington, A. Paton, T. B. Reynolds and Sheila Sherlock, of Hammersmith Hospital, London, *Journal of Laboratory and Clinical Medicine*, 1954, **43**, 880.

The patients were then given an intramuscular injection of hexamethonium to produce a rapid and marked fall of blood pressure and simultaneously they were given insulin intravenously in order to cause a rapid and marked fall of blood sugar. It is recorded that none of the patients became comatose as a result but that 'they invariably passed from drowsiness to peaceful sleep'. Seven of them sweated profusely.

A later report was published describing the injection into the spleen of a contrast medium (50 c.c. of a 50% diodone) and serial X-rays on forty patients with enlarged spleens, which in most patients was secondary to liver cirrhosis. This series included a boy of seventeen and a girl of eleven years. It must be emphasized that in some experiments described subsequently this procedure is merely the first step of a more elaborate investigation. But that even this investigation by itself is not so simple as it sounds can be gauged from the fact these experts failed to obtain satisfactory results in five of the forty patients. In eight patients the contrast medium was inadvertently injected into the peritoneal cavity with resultant severe pain, but in three of the patients, in spite of this occurrence, the procedure was repeated.[1]

This technique was also done on eighty-four patients, sixty-five of whom had cirrhosis of the liver. In six patients the bulk of the contrast medium was accidentally injected into the peritoneal cavity, producing, 'quite severe pain, but in most cases this persisted for less than one hour'. The possibility of some complication occurring at a much later date directly due to this accident, such as peritoneal adhesions with subsequent intestinal obstruction, cannot be ruled out. Moreover, two of the patients had severe haemorrhage as a result of the splenic puncture and had to have blood transfusions. In one patient the needle accidentally pierced the bowel; two others had a mild degree of shock as a result of the investigation, and three vomited blood immediately after it.[2]

Another experiment on patients with liver disease, some of whom had mental confusion, was done to demonstrate whether

[1] M. Atkinson, E. Barnett, Sheila Sherlock and Steiner, of Hammersmith Hospital, *Quarterly Journal of Medicine*, 1955, **24**, 77.
[2] Steiner, Sheila Sherlock and M. D. Turner, of Hammersmith Hospital *Journal of Faculty of Radiologists*, 1957, **8**, 158.

or not abnormal veins developed (collateral circulation) connecting liver and lung veins, as a result of liver vein obstruction resulting from the liver cirrhosis. This investigation was carried out on twelve patients with liver disease, of whom six had neuro-psychiatric symptoms, three of severe degree. A catheter was inserted into the femoral artery to collect frequent blood samples. Radioactive krypton was injected into the main arm vein and the same radioactive material was also injected into the spleen via a needle inserted into that organ. In two patients, in addition, another radioactive substance (H.I.S.A.) was injected into the spleen.[1]

Another method of radiological visualization of the liver and splenic blood-vessels has been described. This entails the passage of a catheter via the femoral artery and so into the abdominal aorta and then into one of its main branches, either the coeliac axis artery, and so into the splenic artery, or the superior mesenteric artery. A contrast medium is then injected into the catheter and eight serial X-rays taken.[2]

This procedure was done on twenty-six patients with cirrhosis of the liver; five other patients with portal vein thrombosis, three patients with a tumour of the liver, two patients with unexplained splenic enlargement, three patients with unexplained abdominal pain, three other patients with abdominal tumours not affecting the liver or spleen, and one patient with a blood disease. The authors mention, 'The technique is of particular value in the pre-operative assessment of patients with portal hypertension.' But a large number of those submitted to this complex investigation do not come within this category and it would certainly be very difficult to justify on this basis the procedure in at least eleven of the patients.

Ten patients who had cirrhosis of the liver (including one aged fifteen) were submitted to hepatic vein catheterization.[3] Six other patients were used as controls. Besides the catheter in the hepatic vein, a cannula was placed in the brachial artery

[1] Shaldon, Caesar, Chiandussi, H. S. Williams, Sheville and Sheila Sherlock, of Hammersmith Hospital, London, *New England Journal Medicine*, 1961, **265**, 410.

[2] Kreel and Roger Williams, of Royal Free Hospital, London, *British Medical Journal*, 1964, **2**, 1500.

[3] E. E. Gordon, Anne Craigie, D. N. S. Kerr, Cherrick and Sheila Sherlock, of Hammersmith Hospital, London. *Journal of Laboratory and Clinical Medicine*, 1960, **55**, 829.

and blood samples taken from this artery and from the hepatic vein. After ten minutes further samples were taken. The subjects were then given intravenously 50 c.c. of a very concentrated (50%) solution of glucose very rapidly. Further blood samples were then obtained from both hepatic vein and brachial artery fifteen, thirty, forty-five, sixty, ninety and one hundred and twenty minutes after the injection of the glucose solution. Such frequent obtaining of blood samples over an extended period is a common practice in many experiments. I am amazed at the total amount of blood loss which many subjects of such experiments must sustain.

In 1962 an experiment was conducted which was reported under the heading 'Estimation of portal collateral flow using an intrasplenic injection of a radioactive material'.[1] The experiment was carried out on a subject with undiagnosed abdominal pain who had had liver biopsy and splenic puncture done to measure the splenic vein pressure. As both investigations had yielded normal results, this patient (a man of forty-two) was regarded as a 'normal patient'. He, and another patient who had an extrahepatic portal vein block, but whose liver had been shown to be normal by means of liver biopsy, were controls. The other subjects were ten patients with cirrhosis of the liver (including one aged fifteen and one aged eighteen) and one patient who was studied before and after operation for cirrhosis. The procedure was as follows:

1. Administration of iodides for three days.
2. Catheter via arm vein into heart and through to hepatic vein.
3. A catheter inserted into right femoral artery through which a wire guide and a catheter were then passed.
4. Dye injected intravenously. Samples taken at three-minute intervals for twenty-one minutes from the femoral artery and the hepatic vein.
5. Splenic puncture done to record pressure in the spleen.
6. 'Arterial and hepatic vein catheters were now attached to a pump so that blood samples could be taken at a fast and

[1] Caesar, K. M. Barber, Baraona and Sheila Sherlock, of Royal Free Hospital, London, *Clinical Science*, 1962, **23**, 77.

constant rate.' Thirty samples from each site were taken at the rate of one sample every three seconds for ninety seconds.

7. Radioactive material was then injected into the spleen.
8. Further blood samples were then taken and pressures recorded in the hepatic vein, the right atrium of the heart and the femoral artery.

The technique of hepatic vein catheterization, previously described, was first performed in 1944, but in this report of the actual method no details at all are given of the patients in whom this was first tried out.[1]

The first report of the injection of a dye through a catheter which had been inserted into the hepatic vein was published a year later. This was done on a group of twenty-five young men, none of whom had liver disease, but who had been admitted to hospital for treatment of syphilis. The report states, 'The catheter could be kept in place for as long as 3 hours without untoward symptoms.'[2]

A modification of this technique whereby the catheter is wedged into a small tributary of the hepatic vein was developed on a group of twenty-seven patients with liver cirrhosis (three aged ten, fifteen and seventeen respectively). But a control group consisting of eighteen patients (including one of eleven years), described as 'a mixed hospital population of subjects with mild or convalescent illnesses', was submitted to the same procedure. This group included six patients with psychoneurosis and five with duodenal ulcers. Furthermore another group of four patients with congestive cardiac failure were also investigated by the same method.[3]

There is another early account of the development of this technique and its performance on six 'normal individuals' and five other people convalescing from acute infections, one of whom was only sixteen.[4]

[1] J. V. Warren and Brannon, of Grady Hospital, Atlanta, Georgia, *Proceedings Society of Experimental Medicine*, 1944, **55**, 144.

[2] S. E. Bradley, Ingelfinger, G. P. Bradley and J. J. Curry, of Evans Memorial and Massachusetts Hospitals, Boston, *Journal of Clinical Investigation*, 1945, **24**, 890.

[3] J. D. Myers and W. Jape Taylor, of Duke University, Durham, N.C., *Circulation*, 1956, **13**, 368.

[4] J. D. Myers, of Emery University Medical School, Atlanta, *Journal Clinical Investigation*, 1947, **26**, 1130.

A later account describes its performance on thirteen patients with heart failure and an additional group of fourteen patients 'without any significant disease' who were used as controls.[1]

One example among many is worth describing in order to illustrate to any medical reader how far removed some experimental medicine can be from practical clinical application. The title of the paper is 'Transcapillary migration of heavy water and thiocyanate ion in the pulmonary circulation'.

In this experiment cardiac catheterization was performed on seven patients with heart failure, including one who had had a recent coronary thrombosis. A control series consisted of 'seven normal patients', but no details about them are given. A mixture of sodium thiocyanate, deuterium and a dye were injected into a main arm vein, except in four patients who received the cocktail directly into their pulmonary artery via the cardiac catheter.[2]

Lay readers may appreciate from this report how difficult it is to summarize medical experiments so that their purpose becomes intelligible to them.

In order to investigate 'The ammonium uptake by the extremities and brain in hepatic coma', two research workers inserted needles into the jugular vein of the neck, the main thigh artery, and an arm vein. Face masks were applied and a dye injected through one of these needles.

The experiment was carried out on three groups of patients. The first group consisted of twenty-seven patients with liver cirrhosis, but no mental symptoms. The second group was twenty-three patients with liver cirrhosis who were either actually comatose or had impending coma. The control series consisted of twenty-four patients with no evidence of liver disease, including one patient of seventy-five and another of eighty-two (both described as senile); and a further two patients both dying of cancer.[3]

In 1961 an experimental technique was described under the title 'Hepatic retrojection technique for studying the effects of

[1] J. D. Myers and J. B. Hickman, of Duke University, Durham, N.C., *Journal of Clinical Investigation*, 1948, **27**, 620.

[2] L. S. Lilienfield, Fries, Partenope and Morowitz, of Veteran's Hospital, Washington, D.C., *Journal Clinical Investigation*, 1955, **34**, I.

[3] Leslie Webster and Gabuzda, of Crile Veteran's Hospital and City Hospital, Cleveland, and Boston City Hospital, *Journal Clinical Investigation*, 1958, **37**, 414.

various substances on the liver'.[1] This necessitated hepatic vein catheterization; the investigators remark, in their report, that 'Catheterization of patients solely for the development of this technique was not thought to be justified. The studies were performed on fasting patients undergoing routine cardiac catheterization who did not have liver disease.'

In other words, after the patients had been submitted to cardiac catheterization for investigation of their heart condition, the team took them over and proceeded to pass the catheter further through the heart and thence into the main hepatic vein and so into as small a tributary of that vein as possible. A dye was injected into these subjects intravenously and samples taken from the brachial artery and hepatic vein. The twelve patients involved were then given an injection of a substance called glucagon and further blood samples were taken from the same sites. The patients had agreed to the cardiac catheterization as part of the investigation of their heart condition, but whether or not they had agreed to any extension of that investigation is not stated.

Three years later two of the same doctors carried out a similar experiment on eighteen patients, none of whom had liver disease. Their report states,

> In most of the subjects the investigation was performed after diagnostic cardiac catheterization, but in others it was done as an elective procedure. The nature of the procedure was carefully explained to all the volunteers.

But from the above quotation it would appear that the experimenters had departed from their view reported in the previous experiment, namely, 'Catherization of patients solely for the development of this technique was not thought to be justified.' Furthermore, it is not clear whether or not 'volunteers' refers only to the non-cardiac patients. Of the ten patients with heart disease, six were between twelve and seventeen. Of the eight non-cardiac cases, one was aged seventy-four and suffering from anaemia following the surgical removal of his stomach and another was a girl with a gynaecological disorder.

[1] Russel Rees, J. S. Cameron and A. M. Johnson, of Guy's Hospital, London, *Lancet*, 1961, **2**, 804.

All the subjects were submitted to hepatic vein catheterization via an arm vein and heart, and had a catheter inserted into their brachial artery. Either glucagon or insulin (both secretions of the sweetbread or pancreas) were then injected through the catheter which was wedged in a small hepatic vein tributary, 'almost to the right border of the liver'. In addition, five of the patients had a contrast medium injected through the catheter and serial X-rays taken so that the liver circulation could be visualized.[1]

Some cardiologists developed a technique for the detection and estimation of the severity of aortic valve leak. This involved passing a catheter with a wire guide into the femoral artery and the aorta as far as the aortic valve and injecting a dye through the catheter. This was performed on twenty-six patients with aortic valve disease, but also on seven patients who had no such disease, who were used as controls. No further details about this group is given.[2]

In order to devise a new means of testing the competency of heart valves, two physicians performed cardiac catheterization on twenty patients with valvular lesions. In addition they were fitted with a face mask through which they were given oxygen. A dye was injected through the catheter into either the right atrium of the heart or the main pulmonary artery. But the experimental investigation was also performed on thirty-five other patients who did not have valvular heart disease. Eighteen of these had high blood pressure, nine coronary heart disease, and six had thyrotoxicosis, a condition which is invariably associated with marked apprehension.[3]

A group of physicians decided to investigate the 'Effects of posture on blood flow in the inferior vena cava' and as subjects chose fifteen patients with a variety of diseases. Cardiac catheterization was done under X-ray control and the catheter was passed through the heart into the lowermost part of the inferior vena cava. After preliminary estimations, the patients were tilted, a radioactive material was injected through the catheter

[1] J. S. Cameron and J. Russell Rees, of Guy's and Westminster Hospitals, London, *Clinical Science.* 1964, **27**, 67.
[2] Braunwald and A. G. Morrow, of National Heart Hospital, Bethseda, *Circulation*, 1958, **17**, 505.
[3] Korner and Shillingford, of Hammersmith Hospital, London, *Clinical Science*, 1955, **14**, 553.

and the estimations were repeated.[1] The report states that the procedure was explained to the patients and that their consent was obtained.

A group of physicians decided to reinvestigate the effects of 'measured exercise' on the heart by using recent sophisticated techniques. A catheter was passed via a main limb artery into the ascending aorta and was then directed into the orifice of a main coronary artery. A contrast medium injected through the catheter allowed serial X-rays to be taken so that the coronary circulation could be visualized. The patients were then submitted to vigorous exercise on a bicycle. An electrocardiographic tracing was taken continuously throughout the proceedings, and the coronary angiography was repeated. The combined records from the electrocardiography and coronary angiography demonstrated the effect of exercise on the patients' hearts.[2]

This procedure was carried out on twenty-five patients with mild, eleven patients with moderate, and eight patients with severe coronary disease. But in addition a control series of twenty-five patients who did not have heart disease and whose ages ranged from fourteen to sixty-two were submitted to this complex investigation. No details apart from age are given concerning these controls.

Regarding the amount of exercise which the patients had to undertake the authors make the following comment:

> Exercise was discontinued when pain, serious arythmia, or electrocardiographic evidence of marked ischaemia (lack of adequate blood supply to the heart) developed or when extreme fatigue precluded further testing.

The following experiment was undertaken in order to study the effects of a drug called hypertensin on systemic and pulmonary circulation.[3] Seven 'normal' patients, free from heart or lung disease, one of whom was sixteen, were chosen as subjects. It is recorded that ten studies were made on these seven subjects.

[1] Pentecost, D. W. Irving and Shillingford, of Hammersmith Hospital, London, *Clinical Science*, 1963, **24**, 149.
[2] W. Likoff, Kasparian, B. L. Segal, Harris Forman and Paul Novak, of Hahnemann Hospital, Philadelphia, Pa., *American Journal Cardiology*, 1966, **18**, 160.
[3] N. Segel, P. Harris and J. M. Bishop, of Queen Elizabeth Hospital, Birmingham, England, *Clinical Science*, 1961, **20**, 49.

What is Being Done

A catheter was passed into the heart and then through the heart into a lung artery so as to obstruct its flow. In five of the patients a second catheter was passed via a vein in the opposite arm into the right side of the heart, where it was kept. A wide-bore needle was inserted into the main artery of the arm and the drug hypertensin, which is an extremely potent substance, was injected intravenously. The effects of hypertensin are to raise the blood pressure, produce a marked increase in the heart rate and a fall in the heart output. Throughout the experiment the patients wore tightly fitting face masks with nose clips. Four of the patients were also given another drug, atropine, after the hypertensin and its effects on circulation were studied.

In 1951 there was reported a most unusual experiment on twenty-four patients about whom no details are given except that they did not have a fever.[1] The purpose of this experiment was 'The comparison of intracardiac and intravascular temperatures with rectal temperature'.

A catheter which had in its tip a thermocouple for electrically recording temperatures was passed via an arm vein into the heart. Another similar catheter was passed into the main thigh artery and a third such catheter was inserted into the thigh vein. A fourth thermocouple was inserted three inches up the rectum and a fifth into the depths of an incision (one and a half inches deep) in the thigh.

During the passage of the cardiac catheter the temperature was recorded at various sites. Later, in most of the patients, the catheter and thermocouple were then passed through the heart into the hepatic vein and the temperature was recorded there also. The catheter was then passed still farther into the inferior vena cava, where the temperature was again recorded. In the case of fifteen of the subjects a long needle was also inserted into the jugular vein of the neck, just below the angle of the jaw.

Hepatic vein catheterization on another forty-three subjects has been described.[2] Of these sixteen had cirrhosis of the liver, nine had acute hepatitis and four had severe haemolytic anaemia.

[1] Eichna, A. R. Berger, Bertha Rader and W. H. Becker, of Bellevue Hospital, New York, *Journal of Clinical Investigation*, 1951, **30,** 353.
[2] Reichman, W. D. Davis, Storaasli and R. Gorlin, of Peter Bent Brigham Hospital, Boston, Mass., *Journal of Clinical Investigation*, 1958, **37,** 1848.

Patients as Controls

The remaining fourteen were a control group about whom no details are given. In addition to the hepatic vein catheterization, a catheter was inserted into the brachial artery and a long wide-bore needle into the spleen through which a radioactive substance was injected. There can be little doubt that this experiment was not without danger, especially to the patients with haemolytic anaemia, because of their marked liability to serious haemorrhage.

In 1964 a paper was written entitled 'The effects of exercise on cardiac performance in human subjects with minimal heart disease'.[1] The subjects for the experiment were nine patients who had symptomless minimal heart lesions, either congenital or acquired. As controls seven other patients were used, all of whom were without heart disease, but about whom the report gives no further information.

The procedure was as follows. First, a catheter was passed into the brachial artery. Second, another catheter was passed, via an arm vein, into the coronary sinus (the terminal part of the main coronary vein of the heart). Then the subjects were fitted with face masks and made to breathe nitrous oxide. Pressures and blood samples were then taken with the subjects at rest, and taken again after the subjects had been made to exercise. The catheter in the coronary sinus was then moved so that it entered the pulmonary artery. Cardiac output was now measured again with the subjects at rest and then again after they had been made to exercise again.

Kidney function tests, including intravenous infusions and bladder catheterization, was done on forty-seven patients with high blood pressure and a further group of thirteen other patients were used as controls. The purpose of the study was to determine the effects of emotion on renal function. This was achieved by 'Discussion of important personal topics having a threatening significance'. These discussions, which last thirty to forty minutes, took place whilst the investigations were in progress.[2]

An experiment has also been described recording the effects

---

[1] R. Gorlin, Krasnow, H. J. Levine and Messer, of Peter Bent Brigham Hospital, Boston, Mass., *American Journal of Cardiology*, 1964, **13**, 293.

[2] J. B. Pfeiffer and H. G. Wolff, of New York Hospital, *Journal of Clinical Investigation*, 1950, **29**, 1227.

on the kidney and heart of deliberate obstruction to the blood
flow through the superior and inferior vena cava. Catheters
were passed through the heart and so either into the superior
vena cava (the main vein of the chest) or into the inferior vena
cava (the main vein of the abdomen) of forty-nine patients,
about whom no significant details are given.[1] To the end of the
catheter was attached a latex balloon. A needle was placed in
the main vein of a limb in order to record venous pressure.
When the catheter was in position the balloon at the end of it
was inflated under X-ray control, by injecting into it a contrast
medium. The idea was, by this means, to produce a gross
increase of intravenous pressure in either the superior or inferior
vena cava.

It was found that rapid inflation could produce such a marked
fall of heart output that syncope or threatened syncope occurred in five patients before this was fully realized. In one
subject the blood pressure fell markedly and this fall was accompanied by profuse perspiration and fainting. Deflation of the
balloon resulted in 'prompt and apparent complete recovery'.
The following remarkable statements are made: 'Rupture of
the inflated balloon in a vein has not, thus far, occurred . . .
The latex rubber appears not to irritate the vein unduly . . .
Local thrombosis of the peripheral vein of the arm has been
the rule.'

In most patients the inflation of the balloon was carried out
intermittently for periods of up to four hours. In the case of one
patient the balloon was kept continuously inflated for fifty
minutes and the blood flow therefore obstructed for this long
period.

The same authors also record performing the same experiment, with modifications, on a group of sixteen patients in
whom the cardiac catheter was passed into the inferior vena
cava, but above the main kidney vein; and again in another
group of thirteen patients, where the catheter was passed
through the heart into the inferior vena cava to below the
origin of the main kidney vein. In each of these experiments
the balloon was then inflated with the contrast medium. The
authors report that the balloon was often carried forward by

[1] S. J. Farber and Eichna and Farber, Becker and Eichna, of Bellevue Hospital,
New York, *Journal of Clinical Investigation*, 1953, **32**, 1140, 1145.

the blood stream, even as far as the right atrium of the heart. They state 'on such occasions the balloon has to be quickly deflated for fear that it might block completely the flow of blood (through the heart itself).

With a further group of sixteen patients the catheter was passed into the superior vena cava. These patients were mainly in the older age groups, but no significant information about them is given except the fact that they had neither heart not kidney disease. The balloon at the end of the catheter was inflated as previously described in order to obstruct the particular vein and to produce increased pressure within it. These patients, however, had in addition an intravenous infusion to measure renal function and a catheter passed into the bladder so that, besides other changes, the effects of venous obstruction on renal function could be assessed.

It is reported that in some patients the renal blood flow was diminished by as much as 25% by this manoeuvre, and it is added, 'With few exceptions the subjects tolerated satisfactorily the confining and tedious 3 to 4 hours' study.'

A group of American cardiologists decided to study 'Transeptal left heart dynamics', which necessitated the following procedures: (1) passing a catheter via an arm vein into the right side of the heart; (2) inserting a cannula into a brachial or femoral artery; (3) inserting a specially constructed catheter with a 78 cm. long needle attached to its end into a femoral vein and passing it, under radiological control, into the right side of the heart, then manipulating the needle so that it pierces the septum between the two atria and thus enters the left atrium. By this combined right and left heart catheterization 'true pulmonary blood volume' was estimated. The experiment was performed on twenty-four female and eight male patients aged fourteen to forty-five, all of whom had been sent to the clinic because they were found to have a heart murmur. But actually in all of them convential techniques of auscultation, radiology and electrocardiography had proved that the murmur was innocent and of no significance whatsoever. The published account states,

To date only 18 normal subject studies have been done in this manner (by other cardiologists). The purpose of this paper is to extend the observations to include an additional 32 apparently normal subjects.[1]

Another series of investigations exactly the same as the previously described experiment, but with the addition of the passage of a third catheter via an arm vein into the pulmonary artery just beyond its valve, were carried out on ninety-six patients. Most of them had valvular disease of the heart, but a few had congenital heart lesions. In addition a third group of patients, described as 'a few found free from heart disease after complete study', were submitted to this complex procedure. The purpose of this experimental investigation was to determine the pulmonary blood volume.[2]

Doctors from a famous cancer research institute have done a great deal of research on the relationship of immunity to cancer development, and this has involved the injection of live cancer cells into people. It was found that if such live cancer cells were injected (usually into two sites, but often four, in forearm and thigh) into people who did not have cancer, then the injected cells completely died out within three weeks. Actually in a very few cases the injected cancers were still actively growing at the end of this period, although in all cases they subsequently died out.

These results were contrasted with those obtained by injection of live cancer cells into patients with advanced cancer, who had but a short life expectancy. It was found that the implanted cancer cells lived much longer in them. In technical language, complete tissue rejection occurred in three to eight weeks, as opposed to two to three weeks in the non-cancer group. This suggests that cancer patients have some immunological defect. The number of people, with or without cancer, who took part in the various series of recorded experiments of this nature was considerable, at least two hundred in each of the two groups.[3]

The experimenters record:

[1] P. Samet, W. H. Bernstein, A. Meadow and Sydney Levine, of Mount Sinai Hospital, Miami Beach, Florida, *Diseases Chest*, 1965, **47**, 632.
[2] P. Samet, W. H. Bernstein, A. Lopez and Sydney Levine, of Mount Sinai Hospital, Miami Beach, Florida, *Circulation*, 1966, **33**, 847.
[3] Chester Southam, of Sloan-Keetering Cancer Research Institute, N.Y., *Bulletin New York Academy Medicine*, 1958, **34**, 416; and Chester Southam and Alice Moore, *Annals New York Academy Science*, 1958, **73**, 635.

Patients as Controls

The authors express their indebtedness to the many persons who, with no expectation of personal gain, voluntarily acted as recipients of these homografts.

It is interesting to note that a large percentage of the non-cancer volunteers were inmates of the State Penintentiary, Columbus, Ohio.

In order to test the possibility that this apparent immunological defect in cancer patients is due to the cancer *per se* and not their associated gross debility, a group of doctors from the same cancer research unit injected live cancer cells into nineteen non-cancer patients who were suffering from chronic debilitating diseases. None of them did, in fact, develop cancer. The doctors who carried out the experiment agreed that there was no written consent, but maintained that the patients had been verbally informed that this was a cancer experiment and that the injections might produce localized lumps. But it was acknowledged that the patients had not been informed that the injections consisted of live cancer cells, as it was felt, according to a spokesman, that imparting such knowledge would adversely effect the patients' emotional and physical condition.[1]

According to the same report, the hospital executive director said:

They were told that they were to get cells to test their immune reactions to cancer. There was no need to specify the nature of the cells because they were harmless.

A spokesman for the cancer research centre pointed out that in the early days of such cancer tests written consent and disclosure of the fact that the cells were malignant were insisted on. 'But since the years of experience showed that there was no risk, we felt such steps were no longer necessary'.

Discussing this case, Professor F. A. Freund of Harvard Law School, in his Gay Lecture to a group of physicians, said:

Even if we assume with the doctors that there was no increased risk from the use of cancer cells, I wonder whether in addition to risk of actual injury, we ought not to include extreme

[1] The Experiments were done at the Jewish Chronic Disease Hospital, Brooklyn, New York, *Newsweek*, 7 February 1964 (page 58). See also reports of the same experiment, *Science*, 1966, **151**, 636, and *The Saturday Review*, 5 February and 2 July 1966.

repugnance on the part of the subject as a ground for requiring disclosure and consent – repugnance, that is, if all the facts were known.[1]

Professor Ladimer, a New York lawyer, when interviewed concerning the above experiment,[2] said that there was no court decision in America which governed conduct in experimentation which is not for the direct benefit of the patients concerned, and he therefore thought that this case might well provide an important and historic precedent. He considered that the question of written consent was paramount, but that the absence of such consent, as in the Brooklyn experiment, was not unusual. In fact, some authorities consider that oral consent is in some cases preferable, since it does not substitute a piece of paper for the moral obligation to explain the situation to the patient at the level of his understanding. Professor Ladimer expressed the viewpoint that these considerations do not outweigh or even balance a deliberate withholding of relevant information in order to ensure the availability of subjects for experiments.

But were any of these cancer experiments really completely free from risk? A recent report indicates the contrary, namely, the injection of cancer cells into normal people may cause cancer in them.

The experimenters[3] wrote:

We decided to transplant small pieces of tumour from a cancer patient into a healthy donor, on a well-informed voluntary basis, in the hope of getting a little better understanding of cancer immunity.

A fifty-year-old woman developed a highly malignant tumour (melanoma) on her back, from which later spread widely scattered secondary deposits (metastases).

Her mother, aged eighty, consented to receive a tumour transplant from her daughter. On the day of her transplant the recipient is reported as being in very good health and medically appearing to be ten to fifteen years younger than her actual age. The live cancer cells were injected into her abdominal

[1] Reported in *New England Journal of Medicine*, 1965, **273**, 687.
[2] *Medical News* (London), 14 February 1964 (page 13).
[3] Scanlon, Hawkins, Wayne Fox and W. Scott Smith, of Evanston Hospital and Northwestern University, *Cancer*, 1965, **18**, 782.

muscles. The next day her daughter, who had widespread cancer, died suddenly. On the twenty-second day after the transplant a minor operation showed that it had been successful. Later, because of the growth which had developed, a wide excision of skin, fat, fascia, muscle, and peritoneum of the area of the abdomen was performed. On the sixty-fifth day she developed fluid in her chest, due to secondaries which had to be removed. Later she developed an intestinal obstruction, due to a tumour plaque on her bowel, and had to be operated on again. But widespread secondary deposits occurred and it was decided to give her intravenous nitrogen mustard treatment. But this did not halt the progress of the cancer; it made her completely bald and produced severe ulceration of her mouth. She died of extensive cancer after a long painful illness, four hundred and fifty-one days after the initial cancer cell injection.

The great consideration of medical advance, like the consideration of the undoubted difficulty of fully explaining to a subject a proposed experiment, does not, as Professor Ladimer has stated, 'outweigh or even balance a deliberate withholding of relevant information to ensure the availability of subjects'.

II. THE INDUCEMENT OF ILLNESS IN SUBJECTS

There are many important and serious conditions, such as syncope, heart failure, liver failure, and diabetic coma, to mention only a few, the exact mechanism of which is far from fully understood. It is felt by some doctors that not until these basic problems are solved will further advance in treatment be likely. But a difficulty is that to have to wait until sufficient numbers of patients with these actual complications are admitted to the beds controlled by the particular experimental physicians interested in that particular medical problem, and at a time when complex investigations can be conveniently carried out, may considerably delay possible advancement of such knowledge. Therefore, argue these research workers, it is justifiable to produce syncope, diabetic coma, heart or liver failure in patients with or without these conditions, in order that such research can be speedily undertaken. By such advancements in knowledge great good may possibly be ultimately achieved.

With this type of research three basic assumptions are made by the experimenters, namely:

The end justifies the means.

Any ill effects are always transitory.

The experimenter invariably has complete control of the situation.

I cannot for one moment accept the validity of these arrogant assumptions. In this chapter I shall summarize a number of experiments which have been carried out on subjects whose physical condition has either been deliberately allowed to deteriorate, so that their then worsened state presents the experimenter with the particular condition he wants to investigate, or else on patients whose illness the experimenter knows in advance is very likely or certain to be made worse by what he is proposing to do. A simple instance of the first is that of withholding insulin from diabetics, which has the certain and dangerous result of raising the blood sugar content and of rendering the subject stuperose or even comatose. A simple instance of the second is that of giving nitrogenous substances to patients with liver disease, a process which is likely to precipitate a coma to which such patients are in any case prone.

Withholding insulin

A team set out to investigate the liver-sugar output in a series of diabetics.[1] Forty-three diabetics were used as subjects. Among these were one aged fifteen, one aged sixteen and one aged seventy; also one man who, besides diabetes, had a lung abscess, and another diabetic with the very high fasting blood sugar of 440 mgm. per cent (which is over four times the normal). Thirty-nine patients, none of whom was suffering either from diabetes or liver disease, were used as controls, and were submitted to the same experiment. Their ages ranged from nineteen to sixty-one, but no other details are given.

In spite of the fact that, in some of them, the disease was obviously severe, insulin was withheld from all the diabetics for two days, a procedure which would have the effect of making these patients drowsy, stuperose or even comatose and their general condition precarious. All the patients, including the

[1] Bearn, Barbara Billing (non-medical) and Sheila Sherlock, of Hammersmith Hospital, London, *Lancet*, 1951, **2**, 698.

thirty-nine controls, had catheters passed, under X-ray control, through an arm vein and then through the heart into the hepatic vein; a dye was infused intravenously and various blood samples and measurements taken. In thirty-three diabetic and fifteen control patients insulin was later injected through the hepatic vein catheter. Twenty of the diabetics were also submitted to liver puncture, itself a process which, as Professor Sherlock had subsequently written, should not be undertaken unless the patient's condition presents a 'real indication for it'.[1]

Another experiment involving the deliberate withholding of insulin from diabetics for two days was reported in 1952.[2] Thirty-five diabetics, whose ages ranged from thirteen to seventy-seven (one was aged thirteen, one sixteen and two were over seventy), were submitted to hepatic vein catheterization, the catheter being passed, via an arm vein and then through the heart, under X-ray control. A group of fifteen other patients, aged nineteen to sixty-one, but about whom no other information is given except that they did not have any liver disease or diabetes, were used as controls and submitted to the same procedure.

Prior to the experiment the patients were fasted for twelve hours and insulin was withheld from the diabetics for forty-eight hours. Indwelling needles were kept in an arm vein and an arm artery. After preliminary blood samples had been taken from the hepatic vein and the arm vein, and from the ear and the brachial artery, all the patients were given insulin intravenously. Frequent further blood samples were then taken from all the above sites during the next two hours. The effect of the injection of insulin was to lower the blood sugar content and, as a result of this, it is recorded that the patients exhibited 'sweating, drowsiness, pallor, fainting and fall of blood pressure'.

Hypoglycaemia (low blood sugar) even when it is only moderate is always associated with unpleasant symptoms, but what is more important is that it can also produce signs of brain intoxication, namely, delirium, epilepsy and paralysis. Although these severe manifestations are usually only transient,

[1] *Journal of Clinical Pathology*, 1962, **15**, 291.
[2] Bearn, Billing and Sheila Sherlock, of Hammersmith Hospital, London, *Clinical Science*, 1952, **11**, 151.

they are not always so, and an experiment like this one, in which hypoglycaemia is deliberately induced, must always be fraught with this grave risk. Hypoglycaemia at least in the elderly, can also produce serious cardiac irregularity.[1]

A series of studies were made on seven patients who had either liver disease or blockage of the important vein which drains the liver.[2] Each patient had a catheter passed through the heart into the hepatic vein, another catheter into the main vein of the thigh, and a third catheter into the main artery of the thigh. Samples from each of these sites were taken every ten minutes for one hour and then a special insulin preparation was injected through the femoral vein catheter. The resultant low blood sugar is reported to have 'caused lethargy' in all of the patients and more marked symptoms in one. A preliminary to this experiment necessitated obtaining blood samples from a diabetic, from whom insulin was purposely withheld for four days, in spite of the obvious dangers of such a procedure.

Another example of withholding insulin in patents with diabetes was recorded in 1958.[3] Five diabetics were used for this experiment, including one aged eleven who had a fasting blood sugar of 362 mgm. per cent and an adult whose comparable figure was 664. (Normal is less than 100 mgm. per cent.) As controls, four patients with advanced cancer were used.

A radioactive substance was injected intravenously in one arm and later blood was removed from the opposite arm (from one-third of a pint to a pint). All the patients were made to fast for twenty-four hours before the experiment and during the same period insulin was withheld from the diabetics. In the diabetics the withholding of insulin, which, as we have pointed out, is already dangerous in itself, was undoubtedly made more so by the fasting and blood-letting, because they would cause abnormal blood concentration and further disturbance of their already grossly altered blood chemistry.

A further experiment on diabetics was as follows. The subjects were five diabetic patients (including one aged fifteen and another aged sixteen) who are defined in the report as 'un-

---

[1] *Proceedings Royal Society Medicine*, 1965, **58**, 1073.

[2] Samols and Jill Ryder, of Royal Free Hospital, London, *Journal Clinical Investigation*, 1961, **40**, 2092.

[3] Shreeve, of Crile Veterans' Hospital, Cleveland, *Journal Clinical Investigation*, 1958, **37**, 999, 1006.

controlled diabetics with ketosis'.[1] The subjects were all made to fast for eighteen hours and their insulin was withheld for from thirty-six to seventy-two hours. As a result of this they became hypoglycaemic and the condition of most of them must have been critical. They were then submitted to the following:

1. Hepatic vein catheterization.
2. A cannula placed in a main artery.
3. A dye infused intravenously.
4. Blood samples taken from the hepatic vein and from the femoral artery every fifteen minutes for ninety minutes.
5. Insulin injected.
6. Further samples of blood taken from the hepatic vein and the femoral artery.

Administering toxic substances to patients with liver disease

Patients with liver disease are often afflicted with tremor of the limbs and sometimes with delirium and hallucinations, with epilepsy and with paralysis. These manifestations are collectively called 'neuro-psychiatric'. They have been known for a very long time and were, indeed, described by Hippocrates (460–377 B.C.). They arise from the toxic disturbance of the brain which liver disease causes. But such symptoms have been deliberately produced in liver patients by experimenters whose aim has been, not neuro-psychiatric research, but the production of a state of liver failure in which biochemical and other mechanisms possibly responsible for these symptoms can be investigated. This state of affairs has been deliberately induced in patients with liver disease by administering to them various known toxic substances such as ammonium chloride.

The fact that the administration of ammonium chloride to patients with liver disease produces mental disturbance and tremor was confirmed by Dr. Phillips of Boston in 1952, who concluded his well-known report with the warning that 'the administration of these substances to patients with liver disease may be hazardous'.[2] In spite of this warning, three years after its publication there was recorded an experiment in which the

---

[1] Bondy, W. L. Bloom, Virginia Whitner and Betty Farrar, of Grady Hospital, Atlanta, Georgia, *Journal Clinical Investigation*, 1949, **28**, 1126.
[2] *New England Journal of Medicine*, 1952, **247**, 239.

aim may be summarized as that of establishing that the estimation of blood ammonium values in patients with liver disease is of limited use.[1] The subjects submitted to this experiment were sixty-six patients with liver disease, of whom thirty-three had been delirious and either comatose or stuperose before the experiment. Fourteen of these, who were obviously dying, are described as 'during the last week of irreversible hepatic coma'. Thirty-three controls were also used whom the report describes as 'either hospital staff or patients with heart or lung disease'. All subjects were given large amounts of ammonium chloride and some, in addition to this, were given another nitrogenous substance called methionine.

On the sixty-six patients with liver disease, liver punctures were done and also splenic venography (see page 68). Twenty-eight of the liver patients also had both hepatic and kidney vein catheterizations (two catheters to each patient). Similar catheterizations were done on the control group. With regard to this the report states, 'In the control group the catheterization was otherwise indicated as a necessary assessment of cardiac, metabolic or renal function.' But there is no metabolic or renal disease for which both these catheterizations could be regarded as the usual means of investigation.

In subsequent correspondence about this experiment it was maintained that the primary interest was in diagnosis. The question of consent of the subjects was raised unequivocally by Dr. Sevitt of Birmingham, England, who asked:

1. Did the authors know that methionine and ammonium chloride were potentially dangerous? If they did, was it necessary to confirm the knowledge?

2. Were the patients consulted before substances potentially dangerous to them were given, and did they agree to participate in the experiment?

3. If they did agree were they capable of fully understanding the nature of the experiments and the dangers involved? It would appear that they were not mentally normal before the noxious substances were administered.

4. If one of these patients had died in coma during the trial, would the coroner have been informed and given the full story?

[1] Elizabeth Phear (non-medical), Sheila Sherlock and W. H. J. Summerskill, of Hammersmith Hospital, London, *Lancet*, 1955, **1**, 836.

5. Would they have performed similar experiments on relatives or other near and dear ones?[1]

The experimenters' reply to this was that 'they were capable of understanding the nature of the trial'. But how *could* it be true of those fourteen who were delirious and either comatose or pre-comatose?

When publishing, in a severely mutilated form, a letter which I wrote to the *Lancet* on the subject, the assistant editor explained his reasons for censoring my comments, his words being very similar to those which the editor of the same journal had used to me on a previous occasion.[2] 'I believe there are occasions in medical controversy when the plainest speaking is justified, but I am not convinced that this is one of them.'

On numerous occasions toxic symptoms have been deliberately produced in patients with liver disease by the administration of nitrogenous substances. Some of the relevant experiments are summarized below.

Known toxic nitrogenous substances were given to eighteen patients who had cirrhosis of the liver. Of these patients five had persistent and seven transient neuro-psychological disorders. The other seven were in the terminal stages of the disease and died within eight days of the study. Eleven of the eighteen were also submitted to hepatic vein catheterization. The article reporting this experiment begins, 'Nervous disorders have been induced in patients with liver disease by the administration of certain nitrogenous substances.'[3] And the same article concludes, 'Exacerbation followed a diet containing more than 70 gramme protein (the main source of nitrogen), or containing added methionine (another nitrogenous substance), or ammonium chloride.'

A further study was done on fifteen patients with liver disease, all of whom had had neuro-psychiatric episodes. They were all given nitrogenous substances, as a consequence of which, as had been anticipated, their cerebral symptoms became aggravated.[4]

[1] *Lancet*, 1955, **1**, 1023.
[2] Page 3.
[3] Sheila Sherlock, W. H. J. Summerskill, L. P. White and Elizabeth Phear, *Lancet*, 1954, **2**, 453.
[4] W. H. J. Summerskill, Esther Davidson, Sheila Sherlock and Steiner, of Hammersmith Hospital, London, *Quarterly Journal of Medicine*, 1956, **25**, 245.

A similar experiment was also done on thirty-eight patients with cirrhosis of the liver, of whom three were comatose and two had gross disturbances of consciousness prior to the experiment, the aim of which was to study blood pyruvic levels in patients with liver disease of various degrees of severity. To further this study ten of the patients were given large doses of ammonium chloride, resulting in the expected aggravation of their condition.[1]

In another experiment fifty-four patients were submitted to hepatic vein catheterization by the usual technique, and nine of them also had a catheter passed into the main kidney vein to estimate its blood flow. Twenty-nine of the patients had liver cirrhosis, ten of whom had had previous bouts of delirium. Four of them actually had mental confusion at the time of the experiment. Six of the patients had moderate or severe viral hepatitis, and on two of them the experiment was repeated during their convalescence. Six of the subjects had either chronic pulmonary or heart disease. Five were members of the hospital staff, but their status is not given. Two had jaundice due to cancer. Two had severe renal disease, one of whom had a blood urea of ten times the normal, indicating that he was in the terminal phases of the disease, which is then invariably accompanied by disorders of consciousness. Two of the patients had enlargement of their spleen and liver, the cause of which is not given. One patient had abdominal tuberculosis.

After samples of blood had been taken from an arm vein and the hepatic vein, and in nine patients also from the renal vein, all the fifty-four subjects, except three, were given a large dose of ammonium chloride to study their 'ammonium tolerance'. The report adds, 'The ammonium chloride almost invariably provoked nausea, rarely vomiting.' Then further blood samples were taken from the previously mentioned sites thirty, sixty and one hundred and twenty minutes after the drug had been administered. The report adds that in the two patients with renal disease and in one of the cirrhotic patients blood samples were taken from the hepatic vein, 'every half to two hours throughout the day'. Presumably the catheter in the liver was left *in situ* throughout the whole day. In the other subjects the

[1] A. M. Dawson, de Groote, W. S. Rosenthal and Sheila Sherlock, of Hammersmith Hospital, London, *Lancet*, 1957, 1, 392.

experiment lasted for between three and four hours.[1] All four of the patients who were actually confused at the beginning of the experiment, and eleven other of the patients with liver cirrhosis, showed deterioration of their mental condition as a result of the ammonium chloride administration. One of the patients with virus hepatitis developed a tremor of his limbs as a result of the ammonium chloride and this lasted for three days.

In another paper[2] (in which are cited five reports by different workers who had shown that the administration of the nitrogenous substance methionine to patients with liver disease caused a deterioration in their condition) an experiment is described in which the purpose was 'an investigation into the mechanism by which the toxicity is produced'. For this experiment twenty-eight patients with liver disease were used, nine of whom had had previous episodes of coma. The experiment was also carried out on twelve control patients who were free from liver disease, but about whom no further information is given. Nine of the cirrhotic patients had previously had splenic venography.

Methionine was given orally to all the patients with the exception of eleven who were too ill to swallow. To these eleven the methionine was administered intravenously. Seven of these deteriorated as a result of the administration, four lapsing into coma and the other three becoming stuperose. In the case of four patients who deteriorated after receiving the methionine *orally*, further deterioration was deliberately produced by giving additional methionine intravenously.

The report states that 'methionine was given with their consent and co-operation as a part of a necessary assessment of their mental and neurological condition'. But it is impossible to accept the plea of 'necessary assessment' in the case of the liver patients used in this experiment as their diagnosis was not in any doubt, and the clearly stated purpose of the experiment was to investigate the mechanism of methionine toxicity.

A further sixty-two patients with liver disease were investigated, of whom the very significant admission is made in the

[1] L. P. White, Elizabeth Phear, W. H. J. Summerskill and Marjorie Cole, of Hammersmith Hospital, London, *Journal of Clinical Investigation*, 1955, **34**, 158.

[2] Elizabeth Phear, Ruebner, Sheila Sherlock and W. H. J. Summerskill, of Hammersmith Hospital, London, *Clinical Science*, 1956, **15**, 93.

report that 'the diagnosis was usually evident on clinical and biochemical grounds, but, when necessary, was confirmed by liver puncture'.[1] Nevertheless, these patients were submitted to splenic venography, and they were then given high protein diet, ammonium chloride and methionine, both substances which were known to have a deleterious effect. A daily assessment was made of the effects of these substances on the patients' neuro-psychiatric state, a part of this assessment being made by taking continuous electrical tracings from the brain. These tracings confirmed the previously known toxic effects of nitrogenous substances.

In a report published in 1956[2] the authors quote Dr. Eisenmenger of Johns Hopkins as having conclusively demonstrated, in 1954, that the administration of a diuretic called diamox to patients with liver disease caused confusion. Nevertheless, their own paper, entitled 'Production of impending hepatic coma by diamox', records a further testing of this known point. Twelve patients who had cirrhosis of the liver were used as subjects and were given diamox. 'Confusion and the typical tremor were not present before diamox was given', says the report, 'except in one patient'. After receiving the diamox four of the patients developed confusion and tremor and two of them showed very marked mental deterioration; but the experimenters continued to give diamox even after this deterioration had become obvious, with the result that it became worse still.

A year later, in 1957, a report shows that two of these doctors were well aware of the toxic action of diamox, as their opening sentence makes plain: 'Patients with liver disease given diamox sometimes develop symptoms and signs indistinguishable from hepatic coma.'[3] The subjects of the experiment reported in this later paper were twenty-four patients with cirrhosis of the liver, many of whom were either comatose or pre-comatose. As controls, the investigators used one patient with cancer of the bile duct, one with acute hepatitis, and one with severe anaemia

[1] Parsons Smith, W. H. J. Summerskill, A. M. Dawson and Sheila Sherlock, of Hammersmith Hospital, London, *Proc. Soc. Exp. Biol. and Med., Lancet*, 1957, **2,** 867.

[2] L. T. Webster and C. S. Davidson, of Boston City Hospital, Mass., *Proceedings Society Experimental Biology and Medicine*, 1956, **91,** 27.

[3] A. M. Dawson, de Groote, W. A. Rosenthal and Sheila Sherlock, of Hammersmith Hospital, London, *Clinical Science*, 1957, **16,** 413.

due to myelosclerosis (a fatal disease in which the bone marrow ceases to function).

The subjects were given large doses of ammonium chloride by mouth and a dose of diamox intravenously. Samples of arterial and of venous blood were then taken thirty, sixty, ninety and one hundred and twenty minutes later from a limb artery and a limb vein. This comprised the first part of the experiment and was repeated four times during a period of three days. For stage two of the experiment the subjects had a cardiac catheter passed (under X-day control) through the heart into the hepatic vein. Another catheter was now passed via the inferior vena cava into a renal vein, and wide-bore needles were inserted into a main artery and a vein of a limb. By this means simultaneous blood samples were obtained for the next two hours from limb artery, limb vein, hepatic vein and renal vein – *before and after* the administration to the subjects of further ammonium chloride and diamox. As expected, many of the patients with liver disease became much worse as a direct consequence of the administration of the nitrogenous sub-stances.

An article published in 1957 states,[1]

> It is dangerous to give amino-acids such as methionine, which are toxic, to patients with liver disease. Patients with impending coma are extremely sensitive to sedatives, Morphia is absolutely contra-indicated. Drugs such as methionine, ammonia salts and diamox are disallowed.

But the author of this advice, together with some colleagues, a few years later performed the following experiment.[2]

The subjects were divided into two groups. Group A con-sisted of seven patients without liver disease and eight who had liver disease but were free from neuro-psychiatric complications. Group B consisted of seventeen patients with liver disease who had or had had mental disturbances as a result of their liver damage. To all of the subjects morphine was given, the effects being exactly as expected – namely a deterioration in their

---

[1] Sheila Sherlock, of Hammersmith Hospital, London, *British Medical Bulletin*, 1957, **13**, 138.

[2] J. Laidlaw, A. E. Read and Sheila Sherlock, of Hammersmith Hospital, London, *Gastroenterology*, 1961, **40**, 389.

condition. Electrical tracings of the brain confirmed this. The report enigmatically states that 'The tests were explained to the patients who agreed to it for the better understanding of their symptoms'.

A group of research workers administered a diuretic substance, chlorothiazide, to thirteen patients with liver disease.[1] Seven of these patients were already mentally disturbed at the time of the experiment. The effect of this drug was to make three of the patients pass into a state of pre-coma. One of them had a fit and two others lapsed into deep coma after first becoming 'very violent requiring considerable restraint'. What bothers me about this experiment is that after it had been found that giving chlorathiazide made, say, three or four patients worse, the experimenters persisted in continuing with the administration of the drug to the others.[2]

In 1958 an experiment entitled 'Production of impending hepatic coma by chlorothiazide' 'was described in which awareness of the previously described experiment is recorded, yet the authors themselves administered this drug to five patients with liver cirrhosis, three of whom had previously been comatose. Three of the patients after receiving the drug showed 'the characteristic flapping tremor, somnolence and confusion', and later became comatose.[3]

A later report starts,

> The oral diuretic chlorothiazide when given to patients with liver disease, who have experienced pre-coma, is liable to bring about a deterioration of their neuro-psychiatric condition.

None the less this substance was given over a period of seven days to a further twenty patients who had cirrhosis of the liver, five of whom received it intravenously, as they were unable to swallow. The main purpose of the experiment was to determine if the mental deterioration produced by the chlorothiazide was

---

[1] A. E. Read, Haslam, Laidlaw and Sheila Sherlock, of Hammersmith Hospital, London, *British Medical Journal*, 1958, 1, 963.

[2] The experiment is apparently justified by the statement, 'Morphine may be useful as a provocative test to assess the liability to develop hepatic coma.'

[3] Mackie, Stormont, Hollister and C. S. Davidson, of Boston City Hospital, Boston, Mass., *New England Journal Medicine*, 1958, **259**, 1151.

due to lowering of blood potassium. Thirteen of the patients had either been comatose or shown signs of impending coma.[1]

As a result of the experiment seven of the patients showed gross accentuation of their mental symptoms and two 'reached coma'. The report also states that three of the patients 'volunteered' to be put on a dietary régime for twelve days, the régime in question being one that contains very little potassium and which was known to be likely to cause deterioration. This part of the experiment is justified in the report as being intended to 'establish the clinical significance of doubtful neuro-psychiatric changes', a statement which I personally find difficult to understand.

In 1960 an experiment was carried out of which the purpose was to study cerebral blood flow in liver disease.[2] For this experiment seventeen patients with cirrhosis of the liver were chosen as 'direct' subjects. Of these seventeen nine were 'lethargic and mildly confused'; six were 'confused and intermittently somnolent', and in their case 'disorientation was usually so complete that conversation was impossible'; and three were 'comatose and responded only to vigorous and painful stimuli'. As controls eleven patients with no liver or brain disease were used and so were eight who did have brain lesions. It is recorded that a number of the control patients were also confused and that, of the patients with cirrhosis, one, who was comatose, was aged eighty-four.

On all the subjects a large-bore needle was inserted into the femoral artery and another similar needle into the jugular vein just below the angle of the jaw. A tightly fitting face mask was applied and the subjects made to inhale a nitrous oxide mixture. The cerebral blood flow was then measured. Later, eight of the cirrhotic, one of the cerebral and eight of the non-cirrhotic and non-cerebral group were made to inhale carbon dioxide, which the authors themselves describe as a toxic gas. Five of the cirrhotic patients, including one who was studied twice, became much worse as a direct result of this inhalation, showing increased confusion, disorientation, dysarthria (difficulty in

[1] A. E. Read, Laidlaw, Haslam and Sheila Sherlock, of Hammersmith Hospital, London, *Clinical Science*, 1959, **18**, 409.
[2] Posner and Plum, of King County Hospital, Seattle, *Journal Clinical Investigation*, 1960, **39**, 1246.

talking), as well as intensification in amplitude and frequency of their muscular tremors. This mental and neurological deterioration was transient in all but one of the patients and he became comatose and died seventy-two hours later.

Other patients from all three groups were given diamox intravenously, which, as already described, produces deterioration in patients suffering from liver disease. It is recorded that one of the patients in the control series developed drowsiness, nausea, and facial weakness, all of which lasted for twelve hours after the conclusion of the experiment. Five of the patients with cirrhosis of the liver and associated neuro-psychiatric disturbances,

> Deteriorated, their lethargy, confusion, disorientation worsened, their dysarthria progressed, and their tremor increased in amplitude and frequency. These changes, whose degree was alarming in one subject, were temporary, lasting from 6 to 24 hours. No permanent sequelae were observed.

The administration of ammonium chloride and other nitrogenous substances to a patient with a critical liver condition occurred in 1954 and deserves inclusion here because of some special features. The patient, an Italian of sixty-nine years of age, had been admitted suffering from jaundice.[1]

It was found that the jaundice was due to cancer of the pancreas and a very difficult operation was performed. This included linking together the main vein which drains the intestine with the main abdominal vein, so that the liver itself was by-passed. The operation appeared to be completely successful. Success in an operation of this kind is a rare feat and the later progress of the patient was thus a matter of unusual medical interest. In order to study this progress the patient was taken back into hospital five weeks after being discharged, 'for metabolic studies'.

When readmitted to hospital he had four episodes, each lasting one to three days, when he spontaneously became irrational, disorientated and incontinent and lapsed into stupor. Such events are a fairly common concomitant of severe liver disease, but, as previously described, they may be induced by the administration of nitrogenous substances.

[1] W. V. McDermott and R. D. Adams, of Massachusetts General Hospital, *Journal Clinical Investigation*, 1954, **33**, 1.

The Inducement of Illness in Subjects

On eight other separate occasions episodes of mental disturbance were provoked. 'These latter were induced deliberately by the administration of excess protein, urea or ammonium chloride.' But whereas the spontaneous episodes were comparatively brief, the induced ones lasted up to weeks at a time. The authors report,

> The episode of May 10 to May 15 was induced by the oral administration of urea and was undoubtedly the worst of any. For nearly a week the patient was in an alarming state of profound coma, manifesting no reaction to any externally applied stimuli.

But from this critical condition the patient made considerable improvement. So, it was then decided, 'to repeat the experiments, to undertake others, including the effects of a diet with large amounts of meat'. (Meat is our main natural source of nitrogen.) This piece of experimentation, however, 'was not entirely satisfactory as he had not properly recovered from the previous episode when the experiment was restarted'. So the physicians waited until the patient was entirely free from mental symptoms. When he was, they again subjected him to a high meat diet, with the result that he again became delirious and lapsed into stupor.

The experimenters say, about their repetition of their procedures, 'The repetition of these investigations seemed to be necessary in order to assure ourselves that these episodes of stupor were not coincidental with, rather than dependent on, the administration of protein and urea.' And then they say, 'We were tempted to repeat many of these experiments but further study did not seem to be in the best interest of the patient.' The experiments were continued over a period of six months.

Two months after these experiments the man died, and the very interesting statement is made in the report that, 'Death did not appear to be related to ammonia intoxication or hepatic insufficiency, but rather to age, atherosclerotic heart disease and possibly nutritional deficiency.' From this it would appear that the enormously difficult operation of removing the cancer from the man's pancreas had been successful. It would further appear that the experimenters, not believing that it could have been, regarded the patient's outlook as an entirely hopeless one, so that if he did deteriorate as a result of the experiments it would not matter all that much. If this is so, the whole history of this experiment strongly supports the case against using cancer patients as the subjects of experiments, because an apparently hopeless prognosis may be mistaken. If it is, the patient's chances may depend tremendously on the most, and on nothing less than the most, considerate treatment.

An experiment was conducted of which the aim was to study the effects on circulation of drugs which raise or lower blood pressure.[1] Catheters were passed into the hearts of three patients with high blood pressure and heart failure and of eight patients with high blood pressure but no heart failure. A cannula was also placed in the arm artery. The same was done with another eight patients used as controls about whom no details are given.

The subjects were then given injections of a large variety of substances which are known either to increase or decrease blood pressure, and the effects measured and noted. Some of the patients with high blood pressure had resultant falls of not less than 50 mm. It is known that strong emotion causes a rise in blood pressure, and besides measuring the effects of the injections, the experimenters made use of the technique of stimulating emotion. One patient with normal blood pressure and two patients with high blood pressure were made to recall childhood hostilities under hypnosis. As the experimenters remark, 'Recall of childhood hostility was more effective than fright or anxiety in producing an elevation of blood pressure in the two patients with high blood pressure.' The general belief of ordinary clinicians is that a sudden elevation of blood pressure may precipitate a brain haemorrhage and that a sudden fall in blood pressure may cause clotting in a brain or heart artery.

Production of syncope

Syncope (circulatory collapse) is roughly equivalent to severe fainting and may lead to loss of consciousness. It is a common condition, but doctors do not understand completely the mechanisms by which it comes about, so a great deal of experimental work has been done in an attempt to elucidate this. It is

[1] R. A. Nelson, L. G. May, Alene Bennett, Kobayashi and R. Gregory, of Galveston, Texas, *American Heart Journal*, 1955, 50, 172.

extremely difficult to obtain a sufficient number of patients in whom the condition develops at a suitable time and place for it to be fully investigated.

So in order to study circulatory collapse it is common for experimenters not to wait for patients to be admitted to hospital in this state but to produce it deliberately. The following are summaries of experiments which involve the production of disease by the doctor so that the disease can then be studied. Syncope, which must be particularly unpleasant especially to all very young and old patients, may also be dangerous in the old, especially if they have diseased arteries. In this condition a cerebral or coronary thrombosis may be precipitated by the sudden fall of blood pressure which is liable to occur with any syncope. Syncope is often synonymous with a transitory loss of consciousness, and I wonder if so-called volunteers for experiments in which syncope is going to be induced are warned that they are likely to 'pass out'.

Two London physicians also investigated the effects of syncope on the kidney circulation. The subjects were four in number, of whom three are described as 'normals', but no further details of them are given. The syncope was deliberately produced in them by the application of tight tourniquets around the thighs, tilting, and removal of blood from a vein. The renal investigation consisted of an intravenous infusion and putting a catheter into the bladder.[1]

In order to study the circulatory effects of high spinal anaesthetics the following experiment was performed.[2] The subjects were nine patients with 'high blood pressure of severe degree', and five controls with normal blood pressure, but about whom no further details are given.

A catheter was passed into each patient's heart and a tightly fitting face mask and nose clip applied. They were then submitted to spinal anaesthesia and were tilted so that the paralysis and loss of sensation extended high up on their chests. The tilting also accentuated the liability to syncope, because of the resultant fall of blood pressure. The authors remark,

[1] De Wardener and McSwiney, of St. Thomas's Hospital, London, *Clinical Science*, 1951, **10**, 209.

[2] L. G. C. Pugh and C. L. Wyndham, of Hammersmith Hospital, London, *Clinical Science*, 1950, **9**, 189.

If, as usually happened, symptoms of collapse appeared, the subjects were quickly returned to the horizontal position and given injections to restore their blood pressure.

No justification other than the experimental is given for the administration of high spinal anaesthetics to the patients with high blood pressure. But, as regards the controls, we are informed, 'The high spinal anaesthesia was induced for small operations, but these were not undertaken (after the spinal anaesthetics had been given) until the experimental observations had been completed.' High spinal anaesthesia for really small operations is a most unusual procedure. Was this form of anaesthesia decided upon so that the experimental work could be undertaken? We are not told.

The circulatory response to sudden loss of blood volume by bleeding was investigated in seven patients, whose ages were between seventeen and thirty-nine, who were recovering from various acute illnesses unrelated to the heart.[1]

Cardiac catheters were passed into the hearts of the patients and after heart output had been measured these catheters were removed. The patients were then bled on three occasions during the next ten days, a total of three pints being removed from each patient. Two days after the third removal of blood the cardiac catheter was again passed and heart output measured for the second time. The blood which had been stored was then transfused back into the patients and heart output measured once more.

Further removal of blood was then carried out during the following five days. Cardiac catheterization was again done, but on this occasion a powerful drug for lowering blood pressure was added to the patients' blood before it was transfused back into them. As a result of this, rapid falls of blood pressure occurred together with syncope. Throughout this experiment a catheter was kept in the main artery of a limb, so that blood pressures could be recorded continuously.

In order to study the effects of syncope on the liver circulation,[2] eight patients (of whom no details are given except that

[1] R. L. Frye, Braunwald and Estelle Cohen, of the National Heart Institute, Bethseda, *Journal Clinical Investigation*, 1960, **39**, 1043.

[2] Bearn, Barbara Billing, Edholm and Sheila Sherlock, of Hammersmith Hospital, London, *Journal of Physiology*, 1951, **115**, 442.

they did not have liver or heart disease) were submitted to hepatic vein catheterization and the intravenous infusion of a dye. This was followed by the taking of frequent blood samples from ear, arm vein and hepatic vein. Pneumatic cuffs were then placed round the thighs of the subjects and these were inflated to a pressure high enough to occlude completely the venous blood flow. After such pressure had been maintained for twenty to thirty minutes (the purpose of which was to make a large volume of blood stagnate in the lower limbs and thereby inter-fere with the return of venous blood to the heart) venesection (removal of blood from a main vein) was started and was continued until the subject showed signs of collapse. Five minutes later the pneumatic cuffs were deflated and further blood samples obtained from the catheter in the hepatic vein, which had been in position throughout the whole procedure.

Cerebral blood flow by the usual technique was investigated in nineteen patients of whom fifteen are recorded as having normal and the other four high blood pressure.[1] In addition to the usual catheter or needle in the jugular vein, and application of a face mask, a needle was inserted into the brachial artery. Then, after the initial estimations had been made, thirteen of the patients were submitted to a spinal anaesthetic and were also tilted. The tilting in this case was marked – to five degrees – with the head downwards. After the expected paralysis of the legs and chest and abdominal muscles and fall of blood pressure with fainting had occurred, the studies were repeated.

The same procedure was done on a further group of six patients used as controls, but in their case spinal anaesthesia was not induced. The use of spinal anaesthesia to produce extensive numbness and paralysis as a preliminary to some purely experimental procedure – of which the above is only one example – is something which would be very difficult to justify.

The effects of induced syncope on brain circulation were studied in 1961.[2] A long wide-bore needle was inserted into the subject's jugular vein and another into his femoral artery. He was then made to inhale nitrous oxide through a special mask

[1] Kleinerman, Sancetta and Hackel, of Cleveland City Hospital, *Journal Clinical Investigation*, 1958, **37**, 285.
[2] McHenry, Fazekas and J. F. Sullivan, of New England Center Hospital, Boston, *American Journal Medical Science*, 1961, **241**, 173.

and blood samples were taken from the jugular vein and from the femoral artery. The subjects were eight in number and included one patient aged seventy and another aged seventy-nine.

The measurements were first made with the subjects horizontal and then again after they had been tilted. The tilting was done head downwards for periods up to forty minutes, until signs and symptoms of insufficient blood supply to the brain became obvious. The authors inform us, 'When any of the well-recognized signs or symptoms of syncope became manifest, blood samples were withdrawn quickly, since experience has indicated that progression to loss of consciousness occurs within minutes; and in fact all the subjects developed syncope.' The risk of such a procedure producing a cerebral thrombosis is considerable.

A drastic experiment, not dealing with syncope, in order to study regeneration of the bone marrow, was as follows. The subjects were two patients, one aged eighteen and the other twenty-one, suffering from a severe blood disease known as acholuric jaundice, which is characterized by abnormal fragility of the red blood corpuscles and results in profound anaemia. These two patients were submitted to a process known as venesection (removal of blood) two or three times a week to the extent of a pint of blood at a time. These venesections were continued until 'the patient's iron stores were depleted', i.e. they were almost exsanguinated. The patients then became 'suitable subjects' on whom the doctors could investigate how the bone marrow regenerated.[1]

A group of research doctors instead of producing a fall of blood pressure in patients, as described in the previous experiments, injected intravenously an infusion of a powerfully acting drug, levarterenol, so as to deliberately induce a marked rise of blood pressure. This experiment, which also included the injection of a radioactive material and a dye, was done on ten patients who did not have heart disease. One was aged fifteen and another nineteen. It is recorded that the effect of the drug was to produce a rise of blood pressure to an average of 56% above each patient's normal blood pressure, and also to cause

[1] W. H. Crosby and M. Conrad, of Walter Read Army Medical Center, Washington, *Blood*, 1960, **15,** 662.

an average reduction of 15% of their circulating blood volume.[1]

Throughout this book I have mentioned possible late sequelae of various experimental procedures which have been either discounted or entirely ignored by the doctors concerned. It may be many years before such damage may show itself, and this applies especially to the remote hazards of injecting contrast media into viscera and arteries for the purpose of radiological visualization. For example, can it be completely ruled out that the injection of contrast media into the liver of patients with cirrhosis of that organ will not at a much later date cause further damage to the liver?

An example can be cited in detail. Thorotrast, which is used as a contrast medium, is a suspension of particulate thorium dioxide, a radioactive substance. It has been injected into the liver and spleen and main arteries, especially the carotid. In 1938[2] a leading article in the *British Medical Journal* questioned its safety, but a report from America,[3] written later the same year, indicated that a six-year follow-up of patients who had been the subjects of such procedures showed no sequelae. But in 1965 a group of Portuguese doctors were able to obtain adequate information about 1,107 patients who had had thorotrast radiological investigations between 1930 and 1952. Death had been due in twenty-two of them to haemangioendothelioma of the liver, a tumour almost unknown except in patients who have had thorotrast injections. Cirrhosis of the liver occurred in forty-two and was the cause of death in seventeen. Fatal blood diseases developed in sixteen. A granuloma at the site of injection occurred in eighty-one patients, causing death in eight and being complicated by malignancy in three. Malignant tumours at other sites occurred in twenty-two. The latent period between administration of thorotrast and the development of granulomata was five years, but this was fifteen years for liver cirrhosis and twenty years for liver tumours and blood diseases, although a few occurred much earlier.[4]

The moral is made plain by many of the experiments recorded in this chapter. The anxiety of some research doctors

[1] F. A. Finnerty, J. H. Buchholz, and R. L. Guillaudeu, of Columbia General Hospital, Washington, D.C., *Journal of Clinical Investigation*, 1958, **37**, 425.

[2] *British Medical Journal*, 1938, **1**, 903.

[3] *American Journal Medical Science*, 1938, **195**, 198.

[4] da Silva, Horta, Abbatt, da Motta and Roriz, *Lancet*, 1965, **2**, 201.

to reach positive results in their attempt to extend the frontiers of knowledge may sometimes lead them to behaviour which many lay and medical people would regard as inhumane and at odds with their true calling. It has been described as 'scientific curiosity submerging morals'.[1]

The danger of fanaticism in research and the conflict between professional duty to patients and the possible furtherance of knowledge is highlighted by many of the examples cited.

12. EXPERIMENTS ON PATIENTS WITH HEART DISEASE

During the past fifteen years considerable advances in cardiac surgery have been achieved. Some experimental physicians consider that the hope of further advance gives them licence to carry out any experiments on patients with heart disease, however fraught with risks, regardless of possible aggravation, temporary or even permanent, of their heart lesion, regardless of how ill the sufferers may be, regardless of the fact that they may even be dying. In but very few of such patients is there any question of operation on them, but they are submitted to hazardous and unpleasant procedures not for their own betterment but for the possible improvement of others. Moreover, it is common practice not to give any sedatives prior to such experiments, because such medicaments may interfere with the experimental results. Some of the most difficult procedures necessitate the administration of a general anaesthetic, although this, even with the most skilled anaesthetist, is risky in any patient with heart disease, and cannot be justified unless it can be conclusively proved that the anaesthetic was absolutely necessary. No patient himself can make such a decision. The decision is made for him by the experimental physician.

Heart catheterization, especially in its more complex techniques such as simultaneous catheterization of right and left heart chambers, and the sticking of needles into the various heart chambers, and the injection of contrast media into the heart and main arteries, all have their acknowledged dangers, and all experts would agree that these risks are greater in those with damaged hearts, especially if heart failure is present.

A great deal concerning heart failure and the response of

[1] A. C. Ivy, of Chicago, *Journal of American Medical Association*, 1949, **139**, 131.

normal and diseased hearts to stresses and strains is not properly understood, and, in order to investigate these and other related problems, patients with heart disease are deliberately submitted to such stresses as vigorous exercises, tiltings, and the injection of drugs with powerful actions on the cardiovascular system. Such procedures, often carried out to the point of maximum toleration, causing breathlessness and exhaustion, cannot possibly improve the patients, and sometimes must be fraught with danger. It is often assumed by experimenters that any deliberate worsening of the patient's heart condition is only transient. But every experienced clinician has often seen patients with heart disease in whom irreversible cardiac failure has been precipitated by some sudden voluntary effort. In other experiments dramatic complications such as stoppage of the heart are fairly common, temporarily reducing the patient to a state of suspended animation. By the triumph of new techniques such patients are nearly always rescued from death by immediate action on the part of the investigator, and such an event is often described by the physician as a transient inconvenience. But some expert heart specialists have a strong suspicion that the effects are not always temporary and that permanent damage may result, perhaps not overtly showing itself until many years later.

Most heart experiments involve the following procedures, which I shall later refer to collectively as the basic experiment: (1) Cardiac catheterization; (2) insertion of a large needle into a main artery of a limb; (3) application of a tightly fitting face mask and nose clip, to test respiratory function; (4) exercise on a bicycle or treadmill whilst all the needles, catheter and face mask are kept in position. It is difficult for a lay person to visualize what all this involves. The patient's face is covered with the complicated breathing apparatus, whilst tubes connect his heart and also the main arteries and vein of his outstretched limbs to recording instruments, so that his position often resembles crucifixion and the apparatus is reminiscent of that worn by an astronaut.

The above procedures were performed on sixteen patients with mitral stenosis in order to study 'The minute to minute changes of arterio-venous oxygen with rheumatic diseases'. The significant statement is made:

One member of the team was made specifically responsible for constant observation of the patient's condition and was empowered to stop the experiment at once if he thought fit.[1]

This appears to be an acknowledgement of the dangers of the procedure.

At a subsequent date the same doctors performed a similar experiment, including exercise, on eleven patients with severe anaemia, eight of whom had a haemoglobin below 50% of normal, and one of whom was aged seventy-three. The same experiment was then done on five patients with thyrotoxicosis, a condition invariably associated with anxiety and undue nervousness.[2]

The experiment was also repeated on twenty-four patients with valvular disease, but, after completion of the basic procedure, the cardiac catheter was withdrawn until it rested in the axillary vein of the armpit, and the patients were then made to exercise again. It is recorded that eight patients were unable to complete the required period of exercise because of severe shortness of breath.[3]

The same physicians in order to study 'the oxygen content of hepatic venous blood in patients with rheumatic heart disease', repeated the experiment on fourteen patients with valvular disease, but, after the preliminary exercise, the cardiac catheter was passed through the heart into the hepatic vein of the liver, and the exercise was repeated. Five patients were unable to complete the exercise because of the distress induced, and another patient who had had a clot in the main artery of his leg, could not continue because of the severe pain produced by the exercise.[4]

The same physicians repeated the experiment on a further group of patients with mitral stenosis and also on two patients without heart disease who were used as controls. But after the preliminary exercise the heart catheter was withdrawn and passed either into the jugular vein of the neck or the main kidney vein, and the patients were again exercised.[5]

[1] K. W. Donald, J. M. Bishop and O. L. Wade, of Queen Elizabeth Hospital, Birmingham, England, *Journal of Clinical Investigation*, 1954, **33**, 1146.

[2] Idem., *Clinical Science*, 1955, **14**, 328.

[3] K. W. Donald, J. M. Bishop and O. L. Wade, of Queen Elizabeth Hospital, Birmingham, England, *Clinical Science*, 1955, **14**, 531.

[4] *Journal Clinical Investigation*, 1955, **34**, 1114.

[5] *Clinical Science*, 1958, **17**, 611.

Experiments on Patients with Heart Disease

The basic experiment was done again on a further eighteen patients with valvular disease, one of whom was only sixteen. But in addition a tube with a balloon at its end was passed into their gullets.[1]

A group of physicians, in order to investigate 'The effects of acetyl choline upon respiratory gas exchange in mitral stenosis', performed the basic experiment without prior sedation on twelve patients with this disease, but, in addition, a second heart catheter was passed via the other arm into the pulmonary artery. After the preliminary exercise, the drug was injected through the heart catheter and the patients made to exercise again.[2]

At a later date a similar experiment was repeated on a further twelve patients with mitral stenosis.[3]

The basic experiment was done on twenty patients with valvular disease in order to study 'The relationship of cardiac respiratory effects of exercise and arterial concentrations of lactate and pyruvic acids in patients with rheumatic heart disease'. In this experiment the exercise was continued for twice the usual period and after its completion, but while the first heart catheter was still in position, another heart catheter was inserted either into the liver vein or jugular vein and the exercise repeated.[4]

The basic experiment was done again on twenty patients with mitral stenosis, one of whom was only eighteen. The exercise on a treadmill is described as 'sufficient to cause well-marked breathlessness'. These patients were submitted to further cardiac catheterization and exercise within a few days of the first experiment. These results were compared with those obtained on submission to the same procedure of twelve patients with chronic bronchitis, and a group of twenty people without heart or lung disease, which consisted of hospital staff and patients, one of whom was only sixteen.[5]

[1] H. C. White, J. Butler and K. W. Donald, of Queen Elizabeth Hospital, Birmingham, England, *Clinical Science*, 1958, **17**, 667.

[2] J. M. Bishop, P. Harris, Mary Bateman and L. A. G. Davidson, of Queen Elizabeth Hospital, Birmingham, England, *Journal Clinical Investigation*, 1961, **40**, 105.

[3] J. M. Bishop, P. Harris, Mary Bateman and June Raine, of Queen Elizabeth Hospital, Birmingham, England, *Clinical Science*, 1962, **22**, 53.

[4] P. Harris, Mary Bateman and Josephine Gloster, of Queen Elizabeth Hospital, Birmingham, England, *Clinical Science*, 1962, **23**, 531.

[5] June Raine and J. M. Bishop, of Queen Elizabeth Hospital, Birmingham, England, *Clinical Science*, 1963, **24**, 63.

What is Being Done

Two doctors reported having done the basic experiment with exercise on a further 229 patients with valvular heart disease, only forty-nine of whom could manage the slightest activity without discomfort, and forty-four of whom were so disabled by their heart condition that they were confined to bed or invalid chair. It is stated that all these patients were being considered for possible operation.[1]

In a subsequent report the authors describe simultaneous combined cardiac, respiratory and renal studies in eighteen patients with lung disease which had produced heart failure in eight of them. The renal investigation necessitated a continuous intravenous infusion at the same time as the heart catheterization. Other substances were then injected intravenously to study their effects on respiratory function. A catheter was inserted into the bladder at the commencement of the investigation and kept there throughout the experiment.[2]

The basic experiment was carried out on eight men with severe bronchitis and 'irreversible obstructive airway disease', of whom six had had cardiac failure as a result of their lung disease. But this investigation was combined with renal function tests which necessitated an intravenous infusion and the keeping of a catheter in the bladder throughout the experiment. The patients were made to inhale various oxygen concentrations to study their effects.[3]

The same type of experiment was carried out on eight patients with valvular disease, but, in addition to a catheter being inserted in the pulmonary artery, another one was passed via the opposite arm and made to enter the coronary sinus of the heart. The patients were then exercised for ten minutes with both catheters in position.[4]

The basic experiment with exercise was performed on six patients with heart disease but not cardiac failure; a further group of fourteen patients with thyrotoxicosis but not heart

[1] J. M. Bishop and O. L. Wade, of Queen Elizabeth Hospital, Birmingham, England, *Clinical Science*, 1963, **24,** 391.

[2] Aber, Bayley and J. M. Bishop, of Queen Elizabeth Hospital, Birmingham, England, *Clinical Science*, 1963, **25,** 159.

[3] Aber, A. M. Harris and J. M. Bishop, of Queen Elizabeth Hospital, Birmingham, England, *Clinical Science*, 1964, **26,** 133.

[4] P. Harris, Howel Jones, Mary Bateman, Chlouveraki and Josephine Gloster, of Queen Elizabeth Hospital, Birmingham, England, *Clinical Science*, 1964, **26,** 145.

Experiments on Patients with Heart Disease

failure; and a final group of seven patients with thyrotoxicosis complicated by heart failure. Thyrotoxicosis is a condition due to overaction of the thyroid gland and is invariably associated with undue nervousness and anxiety. Such an experiment would have the effect of increasing these symptoms and thus aggravating the thyroid disease.[1]

Some research workers reported the 'measurement of segmental venous flow by an indicator dilutor method'. We are informed, 'The opportunity presented in patients who were undergoing cardiac catheterization for assessment of cardiac disease.' After completion of the routine measurements, the cardiac catheter, under X-ray control was passed through the heart and either into the inferior vena cava and so into the iliac veins in the pelvis, or into the superior vena cava and so into the jugular vein in the neck. We are also informed that 'A wire stylet bent at the end could be placed in the lumen to assist in guiding the catheter into renal or hepatic vein.' A radioactive indicator (HSIA) was then injected at very high pressure (100 lb. to the square inch) by a specially constructed mechanical syringe.

The experiment was done on five patients: one with mitral stenosis; two with high blood pressure; one with lung cancer; and one who had a deformity of his breast-bone and fainting attacks. The investigation of a sixth patient is described as follows:

> The effects of the injection spray (of radio-active material) was observed under direct vision (by X-rays) in the innominate vein (in chest) of a patient who was having an open chest operation for removal of a cancer of the lung.[2]

Some recent American examples of investigating the effects of exercise on the hearts of sick patients may be cited.

Some physicians passed a catheter for a distance of about six inches into the main thigh or arm artery. A second catheter was then inserted into the main vein of the armpit and through this a dye was injected. A tightly fitting face mask was applied. The

[1] Muenster, Graettinger, Selverstone and J. A. Campbell, of Presbyterian Hospital, Chicago, *Journal Clinical Investigation*, 1959, **38**, 1316.
[2] Shillingford, T. Bruce and Gabe, of Hammersmith Hospital, London, *British Heart Journal*, 1962, **24**, 157.

153

patients were then submitted to 'very severe strenuous exercise on a treadmill'. The victims were nine severely anaemic patients, including one aged seventeen.[1]

Another group of doctors did thirty-two studies on twenty-four patients who had non-valvular heart disease, eleven of whom had heart failure at the time of the experiment. Four of the patients were over seventy and one of these, had had a coronary thrombosis. Catheters were passed into their hearts and tightly fitting face masks applied. They were then made to cycle vigorously for from six to eleven minutes.[2]

A special study on the effects of exercise was done on twelve patients who had cardiac catheters passed into their hearts, a wide-bore needle kept in a brachial artery, and breathing apparatus applied to their faces.

> They were then exercised on a special machine at the maximum rate at which they were capable, until, by a signal, they indicated the onset of symptoms.

According to the severity of these induced symptoms the patients were placed in two groups. The first consisted of seven patients, aged sixteen to sixty-two, five of whom had high blood pressure, and one had an enormous heart of unknown cause. The details of the other patients are not recorded. As a result of the severe exercise the members of this group, 'appeared uncomfortable and desirous of stopping the exercise, but not acutely ill'.

The second group consisted of five patients with high blood pressure, but all of these had had previous episodes of heart failure. In this group as a result of the vigorous exercise, 'they all appeared acutely ill at the time of the first signal, exhibiting sweating, laboured respiration, and facial expressions suggesting fear'.

The authors' summary is enlightening:

> The study differs from others concerned with exercise and cardiac performance in that dyspnoea (shortness of breath) was

[1] Sproule, J. H. Mitchell and W. F. Miller, of Parkland Memorial Hospital, Dallas, Texas, *Journal Clinical Investigation*, 1960, **39**, 378.
[2] R. M. Harvey, W. H. Smith, J. O. Parker and Irene Ferrer, of Bellevue Hospital, New York, *Circulation*, 1962, **26**, 341.

induced without the patient's foreknowledge and measurements were obtained in resting state and at the time dyspnoea was experienced. Preliminary trials determined that the ready induction of dyspnoea in the type of patient under study, required exercise with maximal effort, instead of the mild to moderate frequently used.

In both groups of patients the medicinal treatment of their high blood pressure was deliberately withheld for a week prior to the experiment in case the drugs interfered with the results. It is apparent from the title of the report, 'Pulmonary venous pressure. Correlation with onset of dyspnoea in acute left ventricular failure', that in some patients acute cardiac failure was deliberately induced by severe exercise.[1]

A new technique for assessment of aortic valve function in patients with mitral stenosis was developed in 1958. An incision was made in the neck over the carotid artery and a catheter was passed via this artery, against the blood stream, into the aorta and as far as the aortic valve. A contrast medium was then injected through the catheter and serial X-rays taken. This was done on forty-nine patients with mitral stenosis. One patient of seventy-four as a direct result of this had a permanent paralysis of an arm and leg, and another patient aged seventy-two had a similar paralysis, but fortunately recovered completely. The authors state, 'Their age should have made us question the advisability of the procedure.'[2]

Hexamethonium is a drug which lowers blood pressure, and its effect on the blood pressure in the pulmonary artery was being investigated by cardiac catheterization on a group of patients with valvular disease, when four of them developed the serious complication of acute pulmonary oedema. This is the dramatic drowning of the lungs with fluid because of the failure of the heart to drain the venous blood from the lungs. The report states:

In each of the patients the onset of pulmonary oedema was evidenced by shortness of breath, cough and mental distress.

[1] H. P. Mauck, Jr., William Shapiro and John Patterson, Jr., of Medical College, Virginia, Richmond, Va., *American Journal Cardiology*, 1964, **13**, 301.
[2] S. W. Nelson, Molnar, Klassen and J. M. Ryan, of State University Health Center, Ohio, *Radiology*, 1958, **70**, 697.

The investigators decided that this was an excellent opportunity to study the mechanism of acute pulmonary oedema. To do this they proceeded to measure the cardiac output and various intracardiac and pulmonary pressures whilst the patients were in this perilous condition. One of the patients was also submitted to lung function studies. Not until the estimations were completed were the patients given a drug which produced a dramatic improvement.[1]

A thirty-four-year-old patient had heart failure following a coronary thrombosis, and secondary to this he developed recurrent episodes of blood clots in his brain and lungs. In order to determine whether the clots came from a blood-vessel in his leg or from inside the heart, it was decided to try out a new technique, negative contrast radiography, by injecting a large volume (100 c.c.) of carbon dioxide gas rapidly into a vein and then taking serial X-rays of the passage of this gas bubble in the circulation. The patient died four days later. He was obviously very ill before this investigation, but the authors do not express any opinion whether or not it was a contributory cause of death.[2]

During the last few years techniques have been devised for catheterization or needle insertion into the left heart chambers, instead of the more usual methods in which only the right side of the heart is catheterized. Often combined right and left heart chamber studies are done simultaneously purely for experimental purposes.

One of the more daring techniques is that devised by Bjork of Sweden in 1953. Usually the right side of the heart is first catheterized via an arm vein. A wide-bore needle is placed in a main limb artery and often the patient has simultaneous respiratory investigations, necessitating a tightly applied face mask with nose clip. The patient is then turned on his face, and, after injection of a local anaesthetic, an eight-inch-long needle is inserted between the eighth and ninth ribs just to the right of the spine, and pushed deeper and deeper until it pierces the

[1] Finlayson, M. N. Luria, Stanfield and P. N. Yu, of Strong Memorial and Rochester Municipal Hospitals, Rochester, N.Y., *Annals of Internal Medicine*, 1961, **54,** 244.
[2] Zatuchni and R. B. Chun, of the Episcopal Hospital, Philadelphia, *American Journal Medical Science*, 1961, **242,** 121.

left atrium. A catheter can then be passed through the needle. The needle has to be passed in dangerous proximity to the artery between the ribs, the lung and its membrane, the gullet, the right atrium of the heart, the inferior vena cava, the pulmonary artery, and the aorta itself. Damage to any one of these could have serious consequences.

Added refinements, with increased hazards, are:

1. Another needle can be inserted alongside the first so that both are made to penetrate the left atrium. Through this second needle a catheter is passed and made to go via the mitral valve into the left ventricle.

2. This catheter may also be passed through the left ventricle and through the aortic valve into the aorta.

3. A contrast medium may be injected through either needle so as to obtain serial X-rays.

In some experimental units it has become commonplace to insert needles or catheters into each of the four heart chambers simultaneously.

Concerning the Bjork technique of left atrial puncture using the posterior approach, a distinguished English surgeon has written:[1]

> In a small series of 24 cases we have noted a number of unpleasant complications and there have been 3 deaths, possibly precipitated by the procedure. . . . For these reasons we have now abandoned the procedure.

A group of American heart specialists have recorded their views of the same procedure as follows:[2]

> The earliest enthusiasm has been tempered by the increasing number of serious complications attendant upon it. Since the needle must traverse the free pericardial space, intrapericardial bleeding and cardiac tamponade have all been reported by numerous investigators. This sometimes fatal sequel to the procedure probably occurs because of . . .
> . . . Virtually all reports evaluating posterior percutaneous left atrial puncture conclude that the technique should be

[1] Sir Russell Brock, of Guy's Hospital, London, *Thorax*, 1956, **11**, 162.
[2] A. G. Morrow, E. Braunwald and John Ross, Jr., of National Heart Hospital, Bethseda, Md., *Archives of Internal Medicine*, 1960, **105**, 645.

reserved for patients in whom the information to be derived is
of immediate importance in determing suitability for surgical
treatment. Because of the inherent dangers, its application has
not been recommended in physiological studies in patients
with heart disease, who, on clinical examination, are not
potential candidates for operation.

In spite of these strongly worded warnings there have been
scores of reports in medical journals not only of this procedure
having been done on patients with heart disease in whom there
was no possible consideration of surgery, but also on patients
who did not have heart disease but were used as controls. Most
of such experiments are too technical to be summarized in this
book.

Two American cardiologists did left-sided cardiac catheterization by the posterior approach Bjork technique on 450
patients with valvular heart disease, of whom 40% had simultaneous right-sided heart catheterization by the more convential
method via an arm vein. There were three deaths directly
attributed by the authors to the procedure. In addition sixty-
three patients had major complications. In two patients the end
of the catheter accidently snapped off during the procedure and
had to be removed at a subsequent operation. In five other
patients with valvular disease the catheters became knotted so
that they could not be withdrawn and had to be removed at
open operation, the valve lesion being corrected at the same
time. But one such patient in whom this accident happened was
a man of seventy-two with severe aortic stenosis. After the
knotted catheter had been removed, an attempt was made to
dilate the contracted aortic valve, but this was unsuccessful and
the patient died twelve hours after the operation. The authors
express the opinion that this death was not the result of the
catheterization and did not include it in their mortality figures.
But, in view of his age, it is extremely unlikely that any operation would have been undertaken if the accident to the catheter
had not occurred.[1]

A group of physicians[2] did complex heart studies on ten

[1] B. J. Musser and Harry Goldberg, of Hahnemann Hospital, Philadelphia,
Thoracic Surgery, 1957, **34**, 414.
[2] Cudcowitz, Abelmann, G. E. Levinson, Katznelson and Jreissatz, of Boston
City Hospital, Mass., *Clinical Science*, 1960, **19**, 1.

patients of whom only five had definite heart disease. Of the other five, two had had transient heart irregularity, but had completely recovered; one had lung cancer; one had rheumatoid arthritis; and one had bronchitis.

The purpose of the investigation was to study the blood flow in the bronchial arteries, which are different from the pulmonary arteries. A catheter was passed via the right arm vein into the right atrium of the heart and so into the pulmonary artery. A second catheter was inserted and kept in the left brachial artery. A third catheter was inserted via the main vein of the left arm into the superior vena cava in the chest, and through this catheter a dye was injected. This catheter was then withdrawn and a fourth catheter was inserted into the right brachial artery and passed against the blood stream into the aorta until it rested just above the aortic valve. With these catheters *in situ*, the patient was then turned on his face, an eight-inch-long needle was inserted close to the spine and made to enter the left atrium of the heart, as previously described. Following the recording of various pressures, a dye was injected directly into the aorta, via the appropriate catheter, and further X-rays taken. That no serious complications occurred merely proves what a lot of punishment the human body can withstand.

A complex investigation on twenty-three patients with valvular disease was carried out in 1961.[1] A catheter was passed via an arm vein into the right atrial heart chamber. A large needle was inserted into and kept in the brachial artery. A closely fitting face mask was applied. Cardiac and respiratory measurements were then made. With the instruments *in situ*, the patients were made to exercise vigorously and the measurements were repeated 'in duplicate and triplicate'. The patients were then turned on their faces and two needles were inserted, side by side, to a depth of six inches, by the side of the spine, until both entered the left atrial heart chamber. Catheters were then passed through both of these needles, so that one remained in the left atrium and the other went through the mitral valve, and so into the left ventricle. With these three catheters in the heart, a needle in the brachial artery and the breathing

[1] Samet, Bernstein and Litwak, of Mount Sinai Hospital, Miami Beach, Florida, *British Heart Journal*, 1961, **23**, 616.

apparatus over the face, the patients were made to exercise yet again.

An additional part of the experiment was the infusion of the drug acetyl choline into the heart via one of the catheters, so that its effects on the circulation could be studied. That this drug can cause either heart stoppage or serious heart irregularity is well known.

The idea of sticking a trocar and cannula (a hollow metal tube with a needle through it which projects beyond it) directly into the left ventricle of the heart was first put into practice in 1951. This was done forty-five times on thirty anaesthetized patients and a contrast medium injected through the cannula after removal of the needle, followed by the usual serial X-rays. No details at all are given about any of the patients: whether any had heart disease or not, and why they had been given anaesthetics. But the authors do make the comment:[1]

> We did not underestimate the fact that the idea would provoke aversion, arouse criticism, and be considered an inhumane method.

A new technique for pressure measurements in the right and left cardiac chambers simultaneously was developed in 1960. Two needles, one longer than the other, were welded together and inserted through the chest just to the left of the breast-bone, so that the shorter needle pierced the right atrium, but the longer one went further, through the right atrium and through the spetum dividing the atria, so that it entered the left atrium. The further account of the procedure is worth recording in full in the experimenters' own words.[2]

> Seven patients were studied by this technique. All procedures were performed in the operating room with the patient under a general anaesthetic. A thoracotomy (opening of the chest) was performed on six patients, and at this time the site of the needle puncture was assessed and the appearance of blood in the pericardial space noted. After the completion of the procedure, and surgery, if any, a chest X-ray was done in

[1] Ponsdomenech and B. Nunez, of Havana, Cuba, *American Heart Journal*, 1951, 41, 643.
[2] Derrick, Eggers, Leonard and Paley, of Galveston, Texas, *American Heart Journal*, 1960, 59, 442.

order to discover a possible pneumothorax, since the course of the needle might, in some instances, penetrate the right lung. On one patient we performed the simultaneous needle puncture of the left ventricle (with a third needle through the chest). On one patient who underwent the study no operative procedure was performed. He was carefully observed for two hours in the recovery room for evidence of cardiac tamponade (increasing pressure in the pericardial space as a result of haemorrhage).

The most noteworthy feature of this account is its almost complete lack of important relevant information concerning the patients (except that one had mitral stenosis) and why they were submitted to the investigation. No reason for opening their chests is given. No reason for giving any of them anaesthetics or mention of consent is even hinted at.

Another new method of simultaneous needling of the right and left heart chambers was described in 1961.[1] A needle was inserted between the fourth and fifth ribs immediately to the right of the breast-bone, so as to enter the right atrium and then pierce the septum between the atria and to enter the left atrium. Another needle was then inserted immediately to the left of the lowermost part of the breast-bone, so as to enter the right ventricle, and it was then pushed through the septum dividing the two ventricles so as to enter the left ventricle. A large-bore needle was kept in the brachial artery. If aortic valve disease was being investigated, then, in addition, a catheter with wire guide was passed via the femoral artery through the abdominal and chest aorta as far as the aortic valve itself. In all cases a contrast medium was injected into the left ventricle and blood samples taken from the left atrium and ventricle and the brachial artery. The needles were then withdrawn a little back through the septa so that they remained in the right atrium and ventricle respectively. Further blood samples were taken and pressures in these chambers recorded. The advice is given 'Stab incisions at each site will facilitate passage of the needles'. Further advice is 'The ventricular needle should not be left in place longer than necessary, as leaving it in the heart wall for extended periods leads to significant trauma. There should be

[1] Schaffer, Lemmon, Herose, Casale, R. O'Connor, and C. P. Bailey, of Flower and Fifth Avenue Hospitals, New York, *American Journal Cardiology*, 1962, **10,** 74.

no more than three attempts at any one session to insert the ventricular needle. The patient is observed in the recovery room for four hours afterwards and is kept at complete bed rest until the following day. Vital signs are monitored every two hours.'

This technique, which the authors called 'ante-thoracic pancardiocentesis' was performed ninety-three times on a total of eighty-seven patients of whom sixty-five had valvular disease, twenty-three of whom were possible candidates for surgery, but no further details of any of the patients are given. Whether or not any patients with normal hearts were used as controls is not stated.

Accidental puncture by the needles of the aorta, pulmonary artery, or parts of the heart not intended, occurred in nine patients. Severe complications resulted in five. One patient developed evidence of coronary thrombosis, during the proce- dure, as shown on an electrocardiograph. It is recorded that he made an uneventful recovery, but, in such circumstances, no physician can be certain whether or not some residual per- manent damage has not taken place. One patient developed rapidly increasing pressure in the pericardial sac due to haemorrhage, which necessitated an emergency operation. It is reported, 'He had a stormy postoperative course'. This same patient later developed jaundice due to a 'serum hepatitis,' pro- duced by blood transfusions given to combat the haemorrhage. He died from liver damage three months after this experiment.

Another patient who had haemorrhage into his pericardial sac as a result of the experiment developed a protracted febrile illness and had to have an operation on his pericardium six weeks after the investigation. In another patient the needle accidentally damaged a coronary artery and this necessitated an emergency operation to suture it.

The authors state:

These undesirable events occurred for the most part in the first dozen examinations. This suggests that we may hope to avoid them with care and experience.

This is but a repetition of a common fallacy propounded by many experimental physicians, namely, serious reactions to new techniques are to be expected, but subsequent practice will so improve the procedure that complications will necessarily be eliminated.

A recent experiment has been published. It was performed on five patients who had high blood pressure, two patients with valvular heart disease, a patient with a duodenal ulcer and another with arterial disease. It consisted of the insertion of a large needle into the femoral artery, through which was passed a catheter as far as the upper part of the external iliac artery. A second needle was then stabbed into the same femoral artery and through it another catheter passed to five centimetres beyond the first, the position of both catheters being checked by X-ray control. With the aid of elaborate recording instruments the pressure in the artery at both sites was measured. Pressure cuffs were then applied around both mid-thighs and the arterial pressures recorded before, during the inflation of the cuffs and after deflation. A contrast medium was then injected through one of the catheters and serial X-rays taken. The procedure lasted from forty-five to seventy-five minutes.[1]

A more unusual technique called bronchial arteriography has been devised. This consists of passing a cardiac catheter with wire guide through a large-bore needle inserted into a femoral artery. The catheter is guided under X-ray control until it enters the aorta and is positioned near the origin of the subclavian artery. A contrast medium is then injected and serial X-rays taken to visualize the arteries supplying the bronchi. This was done on thirty-two patients including seventeen who had cancer of the lung (six of whom were over seventy). One of the series was a boy of seventeen suffering from the serious fungus infection of the lung called actinomycosis, and another was only fifteen with chronic lung disease.[2]

The same doctor, together with some associates, repeated this experimental investigation to visualize the bronchial arteries on a further one hundred patients of whom fifty-five had cancer of the lung; four had cancer of the gullet; and forty-one had various other conditions, mainly affecting the lungs. Six of the patients had the serious and often fatal condition of acute

[1] Gabi, of Hammersmith Hospital, London, *Clinical Science*, 1965, **29**, 45.
[2] M. Viamonte, of Jackson Memorial Hospital, Miami, Florida, *Radiology*, 1964, **83**, 830.

pulmonary embolism (clot in a main lung artery). In six patients the diagnosis is described as 'unknown'.

A justification for this research given by the authors is that it may prove useful in distinguishing benign from malignant tumours of the lung. Benign tumours of the lung are comparatively rare and can often be diagnosed with certainty by the easier technique of passing a tube into the bronchi; even an exploratory operation seems to me to be far less drastic and more certain diagnostically than this complex method.

The authors inform us that this is only a preliminary communication and the procedure was done with a local anaesthetic, but

> We are planning some studies under general anaesthesia. This should permit the use of larger amounts of contrast medium.

These experimenters do admit that 'spinal cord damage is a theoretical hazard'.[1]

13. RESEARCH ON KIDNEY DISEASES

During the last twenty-five years some very significant advances have been made in the understanding and treatment of diseases of the kidney. I would like, in the present chapter, to consider two much-practised kinds of experiments, known respectively as renal biopsy and renal angiography, by which the kidney is investigated, and also the question of kidney transplants.

The technique of renal biopsy is similar to that of liver biopsy. After the injection of a local anaesthetic, a wide-bore needle is inserted through the muscles of the loin directly into the kidney substance and a fragment of kidney tissue is sucked out through the needle. This fragment can then be examined under a microscope. The special risks attending the performance of kidney biopsy are similar to those attached to liver biopsy: haemorrhage, infection, and the accidental puncture of adjacent organs. The authorities on kidney biopsy have pointed out the many contra-indications to its performance.[2]

---

[1] M. Viamonte, R. E. Parks and W. M. Smoak of Jackson Memorial Hospital, Miami, *Radiology*, 1965, **85**, 205.

[2] *Lancet*, 1954, **1**, 1047; *Proceedings of the Royal Society of Medicine*, 1956, 49; *Archives of Internal Medicine*, 1958, **101**, 439.

Research on Kidney Diseases

By avoiding the use of this technique on subjects where any of these contra-indications are in evidence, a few experts have achieved a low incidence of mortality and of complications. Others, however, have shown fewer scruples; many reports have appeared of kidney biopsies done on patients who showed one or another contra-indication to this procedure.

The general risk attached to kidney biopsy is emphasized by a leading article in the *Lancet* in 1955, which comments:

> Several patients have had as many as four successive renal biopsies, giving detailed information of progressive renal disease which could not have been obtained by other means. This is not an adequate justification for a potentially dangerous operation; and biopsy should be used only when the information it gives will be of direct advantage to the patients, and not merely a rather academic addition to medical knowledge.[1]

And this view is again emphasized by the greatest authority, who, commenting on the article from which the above is an excerpt, wrote to the *Lancet* that, 'This is a most important statement, for it emphasizes again that the clinical investigator must first by a clinician, whose chief consideration is the care of the patient.[2]

Sometimes those proceeding with kidney biopsy justify their use of the process on the grounds that it can be the means to achieving greater accuracy of diagnosis. But, as the article in the *Lancet* just quoted says: 'Accurate diagnosis of renal disease is rarely of such immediate and crucial importance.' The reason why that is so is because such refinements of diagnosis do not influence treatment or prognosis.

In a review of the published accounts of renal biopsy the authors comment:[3]

> . . . several deaths have occurred on first attempts in a small series. The natural reluctance to report the tragedy has kept some of the experience from the literature. . . . Complications have been experienced in almost all series.

The same authors point out that some haemorrhage from the kidney always occurs with this procedure. This is usually slight,

---

[1] *Lancet*, 1955, **2**, 1231.
[2] R. M. Kark, of Presbyterian Hospital, Chicago, *Lancet*, 1956, **1**, 51.
[3] J. D. Arnold and Spargo, of Chicago, *Circulation*, 1959, **19**, 609.

but if the needle punctures the renal vein or artery it may be very severe. Concerning this they make the following dismissing comment:

> Many of these severe haemorrhages are self limited requiring only simple transfusion.

But to make only one point, blood transfusion has its own risks.[1] They summarize their opinion of renal biopsy by saying, 'For most patients the risks do not appear to be excessive.' But who is the judge of whether or not any risk is 'excessive'—the experimenter or the subject?

Indeed, a very much less complacent view of the dangers involved has been expressed by an English physician, who has written, 'The kidney is not an easy target.' In substantiation of this view he cites the fact that even the greatest experts fail to get an adequate specimen in 7% of cases. In inexperienced hands such failure rate may be as high as 25%. The lay reader should appreciate that failure usually means that the needle has entered some organ other than the kidney. The author comments:[2]

> It is doubly disturbing that the needle that misses the kidney is in danger of hitting the small bowel or colon. . . . Although dangerous complications are rare, troublesome ones are fairly common.

He also points out:

> Some operators allow themselves 2 or 3 attempts; few would resist the temptation to explore a little deeper each time. . . . Something which may be recorded as a mild discomfort can be experienced by the patient as a severe pain.

This last point is, unfortunately, undoubtedly true of many records of experiments.

Renal angiography is the method of taking X-rays of the arteries of the kidneys. To do this it is necessary to inject a contrast medium into these arteries. This can be achieved either by translumbar aortography (described previously on

---

[1] In America it also carries with it its own extra expense, the patients usually having to pay for the blood received at a rate which varies locally from five to thirty dollars per pint. (See, for example, *Medical News*, 22 January 1965.)

[2] D. N. S. Kerr, of Newcastle upon Tyne, England, *Lancet*, 1960, **2,** 1370.

page 23), necessitating sticking a long needle, through the back muscles, directly into the aorta. Or it can be done by passing a catheter and wire guide through a needle inserted into the femoral artery and directing it into a renal artery. In either case the contrast medium is then injected through the catheter or needle and serial X-rays then taken.

One of the first reports of renal angiography by the trans-lumbar route was written in 1946 and recorded its performance on seventeen patients of whom the medical details are given only for two. The procedure was done twice on two patients and three times on two others. One patient was aged seventy-three and had marked high blood pressure and such extreme calcification of his aorta and its main branches as to render such an investigation difficult if not actually hazardous.[1]

One of the first reports of renal angiography by the femoral artery route was published in 1953. No details of the twenty-six patients submitted to this investigation are given or the reasons for this investigation, other than the vague statement that it was done in most instances to obtain renal arteriograms.[2]

During the procedure one of the patients became hysterical and 'brief psychiatric treatment became necessary'. (The exact nature of this treatment is not stated.) Another patient developed a fistula, an abnormal communication, between his femoral artery and femoral vein, as a result of injury to the artery during the catheterization. This necessitated subsequent surgical repair. A third patient had an abrupt fall of blood pressure, with resultant shock, but responded to emergency treatment. An interesting comment is:

> We did not hesitate to use the opposite femoral artery immediately, if an initial attempt failed. In a number of cases the films were a positive aid to diagnosis.

The time taken for the procedure varied from forty-five to one hundred and twenty minutes.

An authority on renal angiography has written:

[1] F. B. Wagner, of Jefferson Hospital, Philadelphia, *Journal of Urology*, 1946, **56,** 625.
[2] Peirce and Ramey, of U.S. Marine Hospital, Bethseda, Maryland, *Journal of Urology*, 1953, **69,** 578.

Only in isolated carefully selected instances is one justified in using renal angiography as it is often unnecessary and frequently a redundant procedure. Certainly its indiscriminate use is to be deplored. . . . It adds an additional burden of expense and often fails to provide significant information which alters treatment. . . . The technique however provides pictures which are quite pleasing to our aesthetic sense.[1]

But once again we come up against the problem as to what constitutes 'a real indication'. Is experimentation *per se*, that is, is performance when it is not a direct benefit to the patient, a 'real indication'?

An English expert on this technique reported in 1961 having done renal angiography in 260 patients with high blood pressure (120 by translumbar route and the rest by the femoral route) and stated:

The cases were largely unselected and the procedure was carried out on all cases of hypertension of unknown etiology admitted to the medical unit.[2]

The same report contains the following warnings:

The hazards of renal angiography are now widely appreciated. . . . The most serious being renal damage and paralysis of the limbs. . . . With catheterization via the femoral artery a relatively large hole in that artery is inevitable, and great care must be exercised to control postoperative haemorrhage. These accidents serve to emphasize that renal angiography should not be undertaken lightly, nor by the inexperienced.

The same English expert and his colleagues two years later reported that they had done over 500 renal angiographies in patients with high blood pressure and note:

At our hospital we have been routinely investigating high blood pressure patients by renal angiography for several years.[3]

[1] T. F. Nesbitt, of Ann Arbor, Michigan, *American Journal of Roentgenology*, 1955, **73**, 574.
[2] D. Sutton, Brunton and Starer, of St. Mary's Hospital, London, *Clinical Radiology*, 1961, **12**, 80.
[3] D. Sutton, F. J. Brunton, E. C. Foot and J. Guthrie of St. Mary's Hospital London, *Clinical Radiology*, 1963, **14**, 381.

Research on Kidney Diseases

Is it a justifiable routine investigation in such patients? The President of the Royal College of Physicians of Edinburgh has expressed the opinion that renal angiography and renal biopsy are justified only if surgery is definitely indicated by the patient's condition.[1]

A more complex investigation to study 'Effects of intrarenal infusions of bradykinin and acetylcholine on renal blood flow in man' has been reported. The procedure was as follows. A catheter was passed along the saphenous vein of the thigh, which had been exposed by an incision, until it entered the renal vein. Another catheter was passed via the femoral artery into the renal artery on the same side. A contrast medium was injected through the latter catheter and serial X-rays taken. A radioactive compound and also a dye were injected through the catheters and blood samples were taken from the renal vein and its artery; pressures were also recorded in these vessels. The investigation was done on seven patients (including one of fifteen), six of whom had high blood pressure and one had marked protein excretion in his urine. In this last patient catheterization of the renal vein could be justified on medical grounds. But what of the catheterization of the artery? In the other patients catheterization of the renal artery alone might be justifiable, but only if simpler methods had first shown that one kidney was contracted.

The first part of the experiment was followed by the injection, by means of a pump, of powerfully acting substances, synthetic bradykinin and acetylcholine, directly into the renal artery, to study their effects on blood flow through the kidney. This latter part of the experiment, whatever may be thought about the first part, seems to have been definitely experimental, having no considered diagnostic value.[2]

A supposed justification for renal angiography is that it may show abnormal contractions of the renal artery, but an interesting recent publication proves that such a radiological appearance may be entirely functional and not due to disease of the renal artery. In a series of renal angiographies done via the

[1] J. D. S. Cameron giving Williams's Lecture at Liverpool University, quoted in *Medical News*, 15 November 1963.

[2] C. T. Dollery, L. I. Goldberg and B. L. Pentecost, of Hammersmith Hospital, London, *Clinical Science* 1965, **29**, 433.

femoral artery route on 600 patients ('In all but a few patients it was performed for the evaluation of arterial hypertension') such 'functional' non-significant renal artery contraction was found in nineteen patients. In four of these its transitory and therefore unimportant nature was definitely proved by repeating the investigation which subsequently showed normal renal arteries. The authors point out that mechanical stimulation of the renal artery by needle, catheter or wire guide or chemical irritation by the contrast medium, may possibly cause a transitory abnormality of the renal artery.[1]

This submission to renal angiography of large numbers of patients suffering from high blood pressure without any real selection is justified by some investigators in that thereby some cases may be discovered to be due to unilateral renal artery disease which may possibly be amenable to surgery. This is a grossly exaggerated likelihood, the true frequency of such a contingency being very small. Is it justifiable to perform such a complex and hazardous investigation on 100 patients in order to find one who will possibly be suitable for surgery? This itself is a difficult question to which there is no clear-cut answer; there is the added difficulty that this procedure has often been carried out for purely research purposes under the cloak of searching out for the unusual case suitable for surgery.

A recent English review highlights these problems. It gives the details of 105 patients with high blood pressure in whom it was considered that a definite indication for renal angiography was present. This was done by the translumbar route only in three, and by the femoral route in the others. Thirteen did show apparent unilateral kidney disease and all of these were submitted to operation. But only three were improved by operation. The authors comment:

> More disturbing was the finding that the investigation or subsequent surgical intervention was temporarily or permanently actually detrimental in a large (21.9%) number of patients. . . . Complications were frequent (12.4%).

They further add:

> Death, paralysis and amputation of legs, and other serious

[1] J. F. Meaney and E. Buonocore, of Cleveland Clinic Foundation, Ohio, *Radiology*, 1966, **86**, 41.

complications have all been described following aortic cathe-terization, often enough to justify the investigation only when it gives information essential for the patient's welfare. . . . The results reveal a morbidity both for aortography and subsequent operation of such proportion as to make it, in our opinion, too high a price to pay for the occasional hypertensive patient.[1]

A procedure which has received a great deal of lay publicity of recent years, but of which the relevant facts have not, in my opinion, really been put before the public, is that of kidney transplants. About this I am more than a little worried.

A man who is a relative, or a friend, or even a slight acquain-tance of another man who is dying of kidney disease, if asked to give one of his own kidneys so that a life can be saved, may feel that it is wrong or callous to refuse. As we know, quite a number of people have been generous enough and courageous enough to say 'yes' to such a request. Or, knowing the need, several have come forward and volunteered to give a kidney, and a transplant has been done.

Many such instances have received wide publicity.

What are the facts?

First, the risks to the donor. He has lost a valuable spare part and consequently his own life expectancy may be con-siderably reduced. If he himself subsequently falls victim to a kidney infection his own life is likely to be in jeopardy.[2]

Against this, the chances of saving the life of the recipient are very, very small.

The reason for the failures is intimately bound up with the still unsolved problem of why the body rejects transplants of someone else's tissue. I myself believe that the solution of this problem will come from immunological research workers, many of whom are not doctors, and not from the surgeons. Until such a solution is found, the obligation of the doctors con-cerned is to be scrupulous in their explanation to any proposed donor of a kidney. He should be told the probable and possible effects on himself and the truth regarding the likelihood of real success in saving the recipient. It seems doubtful whether this obligation is always fulfilled at present.

[1] M. J. Chamberlain and J. A. Gleeson, of Westminster Hospital, London, *Lancet*, 1965, 1, 619.
[2] A case of this kind is described in a letter to *Lancet*, 1963, 1, 1541.

What is Being Done

The public is, in any case, entitled to be better informed than is, I think, the case at present regarding actual figures of success and failure in the matter of kidney transplants. The following figures are relevant. A leading world expert on kidney transplantation has expressed his opinion:[1]

> In the enthusiasm for the great progress being made in kidney homotransplantation there is a tendency to lose sight of the fact that of the 211 non-twin graft recipients only 6 have survived for more than a year.

This is endorsed by an English report describing a series of seven patients on whom an attempt had been made in various ways to modify their reaction to the kidney transplated into them. Only two survived for more than a few days. Of the seven donors, one, who was related to the recipient, was only seventeen, and three of the others were completely unrelated.[2]

This use of a donor who is not a close relative has been advised against on ethical grounds by a British surgeon who has discussed this problem.[3] The American expert previously quoted published the results of his surgical team's experience of renal transplantation done during the previous four years.[4] Six out of the eighteen donors were unrelated infants, of whom three were hydrocephalics ('water on the brain'). This seemed to me to be so unusual that I wrote to the senior author and he replied:

> To clarify some of our donors, most emphatically we never use mentally defective children. The neurosurgeons at The Children's Hospital perform an elective nephrectomy on their hydrocephalic children with internal shunts to correct the internal hydrocephalus. Rather than have the kidney be discarded, we utilize it in transplantation.[5]

It is also of interest that the removal of a healthy organ from

[1] J. Murray, of Peter Bent Brigham Hospital, Boston, Mass., *Medical News*, 8 November 1963.

[2] Shackman, Dempster and Wrong, of Hammersmith Hospital, London, *British Journal of Urology*, 1963, **35,** 222.

[3] Woodruff, of Edinburgh Royal Infirmary, Scotland, *British Medical Journal*, 1964, **1,** 1457.

[4] J. E. Murray, J. P. Merrill, Dammin, Dealey, Alexandre and J. H. Harris, of Peter Bent Brigham Hospital, Boston, Mass., *Annals of Surgery*, 1962, **156,** 337.

[5] Personal letter to me dated 7 September 1965 from J. E. Murray.

a healthy person is illegal unless the donor is over twenty-one. This came to light recently when a woman was to receive a kidney (but subsequently did not), the donor of which was to have been her fifteen-year-old sister.[1] The legal aspect of removing organs from the body is perhaps particularly relevant to a different kind of transplantation which has been very much less publicized than that from healthy donors. I refer to transplantation from patients who have recently died.

In 1963 the *British Medical Journal* reported the following case:

> A man named John Potter received multiple injuries in a street brawl on June 16, 1963, and was admitted to Newcastle General Hospital. Fourteen hours later he died. As soon as breathing stopped it was restored by artificial respiration, after twenty-four hours of which one of the man's kidneys was removed in order to be used for a transplant. When the kidney had been taken the artificial respiration was turned off, the man now, so to speak, dying a second and final death. Before the removal of the kidney consent had been asked of, and given by, the man's wife. The coroner concerned with the case said that he had also been asked for consent – which he had given – to the removal of the kidney, but had understood that this would be done after the man's death. He also remarked that he now considered Mr. Potter to have been alive when the kidney was taken; but he did not consider that any offence had been committed by the doctors. A doctor from the hospital is reported to have said that Mr. Potter was medically dead on the 16th of June and legally dead on the 17th of June.

The comment of the legal correspondent of the *British Medical Journal* was:

> It would be unfortunate if reports of this inquest in the popular press disseminated the idea that there is any difference between death in medicine and death in law . . . To hasten the death of a person whose death (from previous sickness or injury) is inevitable is homicide in law. It is a question of fact whether death was caused by the previous sickness or injury or by the later injury. Anyone removing organs from an

---

[1] The legal problem concerning minors acting as donors for organ transplantation is discussed fully in a paper by Professor W. J. Curran, of Boston University, Mass., in *New York University Law Review*, 1959, **34**, 891.

apparently inanimate body (for instance, one retrieved from a serious traffic accident) must first ask himself whether he can positively pronounce the body dead.

One may say in general, as with other departments of research, that while the experimenters' desire to extend medical knowledge is entirely admirable, the *speed* with which they try to achieve this end is sometimes greater than consideration of the general well-being of their subjects would indicate as safe.

With all this kidney research, and indeed with much of experimental medicine, there undoubtedly is the possible conflict between the seeking after knowledge for its own sake and the immediate interests of the patients. It is important to emphasize that these two considerations are not always in conflict. It is possible to extend the range of knowledge of any disease or physiological process whilst at the same time giving thereby immediate help to the patients who are the subjects of the experiments.

A great deal of medical research is neither definitely black nor white, neither definitely ethically wrong or definitely right, but grey, befogged with this conflict between advancement of knowledge and the patients' rights and immediate needs. My plea is that in these circumstances ethical considerations must be the guiding light when attempt is made, as it should be, to resolve that conflict.

14. EXPERIMENTS IN WHICH NEW DRUGS ARE TESTED

New drugs are continually being evolved in considerable numbers all of which, by law in America and by a working consent of their manufacturers in this country, must be tested very extensively before being put into general use. The Food and Drug Administration of the U.S. Government has recently published regulations extending its already considerable control of the American pharmaceutical industry. American manufacturers are now required to review every drug marketed since 1938 and to show that it is not only safe but effective. According to a report published in the *Observer* in 1964, some American drug firms are, as a result, planning 'to expand their research work in Britain and western Europe.'[1] In Britain the review of

[1] *Observer* (London), 5 January 1964.

what constitutes a safe and effective drug – and one, therefore, which it is ethical to market – is generally a matter of voluntary co-operation between the pharmaceutical manufacturers and the Government-sponsored Dunlop Committee. What concerns us here, however, is not so much the *marketing* of drugs, vital as that question is, but the means by which drugs are investigated long before marketing is approached.

Morton Mintz in *The Therapeutic Nightmare*, published by Houghton Mifflin Co. of Boston, has described legal actions taken by individual Americans against drug companies for damages caused by the administration of their products. Some interesting examples quoted are:

(1) The award of 334,000 dollars (about £120,000) to a woman who had sustained severe bone-marrow damage as a consequence of taking an antibiotic. She recovered from this very serious complication (aplastic anaemia), but the male hormone treatment used to achieve this recovery made her masculine.

(2) The drug MER/29 was introduced to lower blood cholesterol (claimed to be important in the causation of high blood pressure). It is reported that, thanks to vigorous sales promotion, nearly half a million people took the drug before its toxic effects were fully realized. It produced cataracts, baldness, severe skin reactions, and sexual depression. The firm involved was fined 80,000 dollars (about £28,600) by a Washington District Court for withholding and falsifying test data. A group of 175 lawyers are reputed to be still suing for damages on behalf of many clients who claim to have been adversely affected by the drug.

However, I would like to stress that whereas the ethics of drug trials are often discussed both in the medical and the lay press, the problem is neither so acute, nor even, perhaps, so important, as that of research in other branches of medicine.

Many new drugs are, and all new drugs should be, tried out on animals before they are administered to human subjects. But when this has been done it is surely proper for the experimenter to use only the informed volunteer as his subject and not to take advantage of hospital patients whether or not the expected effects of the drug are related to the disease from which those patients are suffering. When I say 'take advantage', I mean, of course, administer the drug without frankly telling the patients that what they are volunteering for, if they do volunteer, is a 'drug trial' of which the full effects cannot be forecast, and also frankly telling them whether or not the hoped-for beneficial results of the drug can benefit *them*. In the following examples of drug-testing the question of consent is mentioned only in one, where the report says that 'the nature of the experiment was explained and written consent obtained', though the possible effects of the drug bore no relation to the patients' conditions. In the other cases the reader of the published articles is left to form his or her own opinion as to whether consent was asked for at all and, if it was, in what terms.

A group of physicians wished to investigate the effects of the powerful heart drug, digoxin, on normal people. For this purpose twelve patients, two of whom were over sixty, were submitted to cardiac catheterization. In addition a needle was kept in a main artery of a limb and a face mask applied. The drug was injected through the cardiac catheter. As a result of this two of the patients developed serious abnormal heart rhythms, fibrillation or heart block. These presumably responded to treatment.[1]

A group of research workers experimented with a new drug called Persantin which was designed for the treatment of angina.[2] The particular aim of the experiment was to see what effect Persantin had on the coronary blood flow. Nine patients to whom 'the nature of the experiment was explained' and from whom 'written consent was obtained' were chosen as subjects. None of these had any cardiac disorder, their reasons for being in hospital being respectively: asthma, obscure blood spitting, hernia, neurasthenia, acute alcoholism, bronchiectasis, and bronchio-pneumonia, and two cases who were in surgical wards for observation.

A needle was inserted into a limb artery and a catheter into the heart. Measurements of cardiac output were then taken. The catheter was then made to enter the coronary sinus (the terminal part of the coronary vein) and the patients made to inhale nitrous oxide through a face mask. Further measurements were then taken and Persantin then injected intravenously.

[1] Selzer, Hultgren, Ebnother, H. W. Bradley and A. O. Stone, of Veterans' Hospital, San Francisco, *British Heart Journal*, 1959, **21**, 335.

[2] Wendt, Sundermyer, den Bakker and R. J. Bing, of Harper Hospital, Detroit, Michigan, *American Journal of Cardiology*, 1962, **9**, 449.

Measurements were repeated after the injection and yet again after the catheter had been replaced in the right atrium.

Another group of research workers conducted the following experiment in order to test the effects of the drug erythol tetranitrate, on coronary circulation.[1] The subjects were fifteen patients of whom five (who included a man of eighty) are described in the report as being 'normal as far as their cardio-vascular system was concerned'; the other ten had either 'angina or high blood pressure'.

The procedure was the following. A catheter was passed, via an arm vein, into the heart and then through the heart into the pulmonary artery. A second catheter was then passed via a vein in the patient's other arm into the coronary sinus via the right atrium of the heart. Next, a large-bore needle was inserted to penetrate the femoral artery. The patients were now fitted with face masks and nose clips and made to inhale a special gas. By these means the blood flow in the coronary vessels was measured. When this had been done the patients had the drug placed under their tongues and its effects noted. It is recorded that in two of the patients with angina and in one of the controls 'marked systemic symptoms of discomfort and a shocklike state' were produced.

The complex technique of coronary angiography (see p. 14) necessitating the insertion of a cardiac catheter into the openings of the right and left coronary arteries, and the injection of a contrast medium, has been used to test whether or not drugs which are reputed to dilate the coronary arteries do, in fact, do so and to what degree.

Such a test has been done on twenty patients with proved coronary disease, sixteen of whom had had recent coronary thrombosis; the other four were suffering from angina. After the initial coronary angiography, three well-known coronary artery dilator drugs were either sucked by the patient or injected into a vein and further contrast medium injected into the coronary arteries to see if they had dilated.[2]

A group of Scottish doctors investigated the effects of a

[1] G. G. Rowe, Chelius, Afonso, Gurtner and Crumpton, of the University of Wisconsin, Medical College, *Journal of Clinical Investigation*, 1961, **40**, 1217.

[2] Likoff, Kasparian, J. Stauffer Lehman and B. L. Segal, of Hahnemann Hospital, Philadelphia, *American Journal Cardiology*, 1964, **13**, 7.

pituitary hormone on the circulation. The substance was given intravenously to thirty patients, 'as far as possible without the knowledge of the subject'. The hormone was also injected directly into the pulmonary artery of eight other patients who were undergoing cardiac cathetarization for some other purpose, the substance being injected through the cardiac catheter.[1]

Some English doctors experimented to ascertain the effects of the drug dihydro-ergotamine on pulmonary and systemic circulation.[2] Their subjects were six patients who had already had cardiac catheterization done in order to investigate the possibility that they might have heart disease, but in whom 'this and other cardiopulmonary investigations showed no abnormality'. Two of them had a murmur which was considered to be innocent. The other four had difficulty in breathing, considered to be 'psychologically determined'. (One may wonder, in passing, about the present condition of medicine in which cardiac catheterization is regarded as necessary before a doctor can decide that a patient's difficulty in breathing is due to psychological causes or that a murmur is 'innocent', but that is not our point here.)

The experiment followed lines similar to those of the previous one, but only one catheter was used. This was passed via an arm vein through to the pulmonary artery and then wedged in a small branch; a needle was inserted into the brachial artery; and face masks were fitted. The drug was then injected into the pulmonary artery via the catheter.

At the same hospital in the same year a more complex experiment was undertaken in which all the subjects had a disease to which the information sought was possibly relevant. The doctors set out to study the effects of two drugs, vasopressin and angiotensin, on the circulation in the liver of twelve patients suffering from cirrhosis.[3]

A catheter was passed via an arm vein into a branch of the pulmonary artery and wedged. A second catheter was then passed via a vein in the patient's other arm, through the heart,

[1] Kitchin, Sybil Lloyd and Mary Pickford, of Western General Hospital, Edinburgh, *Clinical Science*, 1959, **18,** 399.
[2] P. Harris, J. M. Bishop and Segel, of Queen Elizabeth Hospital, Birmingham, England, *Clinical Science*, 1963, **25,** 443.
[3] N. Segel, Bayley, Paton, P. W. Dykes and J. M. Bishop, of Queen Elizabeth Hospital, Birmingham, England, *Clinical Science*, 1963, **25, 43.**

and thence into the hepatic vein; it was also wedged. A third catheter was now passed into the right atrium of the heart and the drugs were injected through this third catheter. A needle was inserted into the brachial artery. Each patient now had four things sticking into him. But in addition each was fitted with a mouthpiece and nose clip which were 'in place during the whole of the time'.

Nine of the subjects received infusions of the drug vasopressin. The infusing took thirty-two minutes and the effects were observed (by means of the catheters) for fifty-six minutes after the infusion had been completed, cardiac output being measured once before, three times during, and three times after the infusion. The other three subjects were submitted to similar studies in which the drug angiotensin was infused.

In 1952 the toxic effects of a drug called sodium nitroprusside were studied.[1] This drug was used in the treatment of angina, but its use was abandoned because of its serious toxic effects. The experimenters gave intravenous injections of the drug to thirty patients, none of whom had heart disease, although seventeen of them had high blood pressure. Blood samples were then taken from the brachial artery, and it was found, in general, that the drug caused a marked fall in blood pressure.

The report is entitled, 'Study in Acute Cardiovascular Effects of Intravenous Nitroprusside'.

A group of doctors set out to study the mechanism by which chlorothiazide, a drug used for increasing the secretion of urine, potentiates the drug arfonad, which is used for lowering blood pressure.[2] Eight patients with high blood pressure were used and the results obtained were compared with those from a control series of seven convalescing patients who had no heart or kidney disease and whose blood pressures were normal.

A cardiac catheter was passed, via an arm vein, and a needle was kept in the femoral artery. Measurements were then made during 'a resting period' of sixty to ninety minutes. A dye was

[1] Schlant, Tagaris and R. J. Robertson, of Grady Memorial Hospital, Atlanta, Georgia, described as 'a large charity municipal hospital', *American Journal of Cardiology*, 1962, 9, 51.
[2] M. A. Greene, Boltax, Scherr and Molly Niv, of Bronx-Lebanon Center, Fulton, New York, *American Journal of Medicine*, 1964, 36, 87.

then injected through the catheter into the right atrium of the heart and further samples of blood were taken from the femoral artery. A radioactive iodine compound was then injected through a catheter and more blood samples and pressures were taken. Now the drug arfonad was injected through the catheter into the right atrium and measurements and samples were taken again. A second injection of arfonad was made, again through the catheter, thirty minutes after the first and the samples and pressures repeated. They were repeated again after another thirty minutes.

Now the chlorothiazide, a drug which is normally given by mouth, was injected through the catheter into the right atrium and for the next forty-five to sixty minutes further measurements were recorded. During this period the patients received a further injection of the radioactive compound. Lastly a further injection of arfonad into the heart was made and the original measurements and blood samplings were repeated. This complex experiment must have taken well over four and possibly as long as six hours.

A complex cardiac catheterization experiment was done in 1963. The patients were in four groups. Group 1 – a control group consisting of two patients with heart murmurs previously proved to be of no significance; one patient with mild high pressure in his pulmonary artery of unknown cause: and two patients with slight degree of aortic valve leak. Group 2 – eleven patients with mitral stenosis. Group 3 – five patients with combined mitral stenosis and regurgitation. Group 4 – five patients with mitral regurgitation. The purpose was to study the effects of a drug (isoproterenol) infusion into patients with diseased mitral valves and compare these effects with those in patients with normal mitral valves.

The procedure consisted of:

1. A needle in a main artery of a limb.
2. Passing a catheter into the right atrium of the heart via an arm vein.
3. Passing another catheter via an arm vein into the right atrium. This catheter had a needle on its end which was made to pierce the septum between the right and left atrium, so as to enter the left atrium.
4. Another catheter was passed via the femoral artery along

the aorta as far as the aortic valve and through that valve into the left ventricle.

5. A dye was injected through one of the catheters.
6. In the majority of patients a contrast medium was injected through the catheter in the left ventricle and serial X-rays taken.
7. After basic estimations had been made of pressures in the three heart chambers which had been catheterized, the drug was administered by intravenous infusion, and the estimations were then repeated.[1]

There is a tendency to justify any investigation of the effects of a drug, desirable and undesirable, provided that it is a 'controlled drug trial', by which is meant that there is a statistically acceptable selection of comparable groups to whom the drug is given or not given. One of the possible objections to any such investigation is that some patients may be denied a drug which would be beneficial to them.

An outstanding example of the purposeful withholding of a beneficial drug took place in the Philippines.[2] The authors pointed out that the antibiotic chloramphenicol was then of proved value in the treatment of typhoid, causing a considerable reduction of mortality. But they were concerned with the incidence of relapses and were interested to find out whether or not relapses are commoner in those treated with this antibiotic. During the years 1951–7 they looked after 480 proved cases of typhoid and gave 251 the antibiotic, but withheld it in 157 cases. In the treated group twenty-eight had a relapse (68%), but none were serious. In the non-treated series there were only six (3.8%) relapses, again, none being serious. So the point was proved that a non-serious complication was more likely to occur in patients treated with antibiotic. But the price paid for this information was that whereas the mortality was only twenty (7.97%) in the treated series it was thirty-six (22.93%) in the untreated. In other words, about twenty people died to demonstrate a comparatively minor disadvantage of chloramphenicol therapy in typhoid.

[1] Whalen, A. I. Cohen, Sumner and H. D. McIntosh, of Duke Medical Center, Durham, N.C., *Circulation*, 1963, **27**, 512.
[2] P. T. Lantin, Sr., A. Geronimo and V. Calilong, of Charity Wards, San Lazaro Hospital, Manila, Phillipines, *American Journal Medical Science*, 1963, **245**, 293.

What is Being Done

Retrolental Fibroplasia (RLF) is a condition leading to blindness in infants. In 1942 it was shown conclusively that it is associated with premature birth. The explosive increase in its incidence during the 1940s surprised doctors because from being a great rarity it had become common. What was the cause of this dramatic rise in the incidence of RLF?

In 1949[1] a report seemed to prove that the increase was due to the vogue for treating premature infants with high oxygen concentrations. Three further reports[2, 3, 4] added further substantial evidence for this hypothesis and several of the doctors proved that by not administering high oxygen concentrations to premature infants the incidence of RLF could be reduced almost to zero. But three doctors, in spite of their awareness of all the evidence and also more recent supporting experience[5] expressed their opinion that:

> Adequate controls are needed however to establish such a relationship beyond question. The present study was designed to test this relationship under controlled conditions.[6]

Thirty-six premature infants were given high oxygen concentrations for two weeks, and eight developed irreversible blindness of both eyes and two others had possible involvement of one eye. A control series of twenty-eight premature infants had only low oxygen concentrations and none became blind. The degree of oxygen concentration did not affect actual survival. So, in the name of 'science', worshippers at the shrine of the controlled series rendered eight infants blind to prove what others considered to have been previously established.

---

[1] *Journal American Medical Association*, 1949, **139**, 572.

[2] *Transactions Ophthalmological Society United Kingdom*, 1951, **71**, 609.

[3] *Medical Journal Australia*, 1951, **2**, 48.

[4] *Archives Diseases Children (London)*, 1952, **27**, 329.

[5] *Bulletin Johns Hopkins*, 1954, **94**, 34.

[6] J. T. Lanman, Laren Guy, and Joseph Danus of Bellvue Hospital, New York, *Journal American Medical Association*, 1954, **155**, 223.

Part II

PRINCIPLES

I. ETHICAL PRINCIPLES

Morality rests on what is right in itself towards the individual immediately involved, not on justification by result, even though that may possibly benefit a great many others.

> An experiment is ethical or not at its inception. It does not become ethical post hoc – ends do not justify means. There is no ethical distinction between ends and means.[1]

The extreme instance of neglect of accepted ethical principles in the pursuit of scientific knowledge is furnished by the terrible example of certain German doctors under Hitler, to which I have already referred. What was done by these men is now universally condemned. But what is often not realized is that the over 200 doctors who were named as participating in those horrifying experiments done in the concentration camps and as part of the callous 'euthanasia programme', were not just a collection of conscripted ordinary medicals acting purely from fear for their own lives, but they included many professors of medicine and others in official positions of power in the medical hierarchy of the Third Reich. Furthermore, Professor Ivy, who was the principal medical expert at the Nuremberg trial, has written, 'It is clear that several hundred more were aware what was going on.' The co-operation and active participation of all these doctors was spontaneous when they realized that the opportunity to experiment on humans far beyond normal limits was presented to them. Not one of the convicted doctors ever acknowledged that they had done anything wrong whatsoever or expressed the slightest remorse. A detailed account of most of the revolting experiments carried out by these criminal doctors has been recorded by Mitscherlich and Mielke[2] and it is apparent that nothing of medical value was

[1] H. K. Beecher, of Harvard, *New England Journal of Medicine*, 1966, **274**, 1354. (In this article summaries are given of twenty-two experiments which in the author's view offend ethical principles.)
[2] The English translation of this book which was originally published in Germany was called *The Death Doctors* (Elek). The American edition was named *Doctors of Infamy* (Schuman, New York) and had an introduction by Professor Ivy, from which the above quotation has been taken.

185

discovered. But I hope that all readers will agree that even if something of value had been achieved it would not even have begun to justify the vileness of what was done. *No* new scientific truth could have weighed in the balance against the suffering caused. Yet these professors claimed that they did not aim to cause suffering – that could be left to others – but that their aim was to serve medical science. Their guilt was that they ignored the suffering they caused in following this aim and that they persisted in practices which they knew were certain to cause suffering. And this, though, as I have said, is here the extreme instance of a disregard of medical morality, is not *in principle* different from an experimenting doctor, in a hospital here or in America, ignoring the suffering which he causes and persisting in experiments which he knows will cause suffering, especially when the sufferer has not volunteered for the procedure, but is subjected to it at the sole decision of the doctor.

This is a terrible thing to have to say, but – apart from the fact that many of the victims of the Nazi doctors were inmates of concentration camps which the subjects of contemporary experimenters are not – where can we draw the line between the experiments done in Germany between 1939 and 1945 and some of those recorded in this book which have been done between 1945 and 1966? According to Victor von Weizeacher,[1]

> There can be really no doubt that the moral indifference to the sufferings of those selected for euthanasia and experiments was favoured by a medical ideology which puts human beings on a level of a molecule, or a frog, or a guinea pig. Today everyone is aware of the fact with the exception, it must be feared, of certain doctors who still cannot recognize the truth owing to their special pre-occupation.

The American edition of the book from which the above quotation has been taken, expresses the point cogently:[2]

> There is not much difference whether a human being is looked upon as 'a case' or as a number tattooed on the arm. These are only two aspects of the faceless approach of an age without mercy. . . . This is the alchemy of the modern age, the

[1] Quoted in *The Death Doctors* (Elek).
[2] Appendix to *Doctors of Infamy* (Schuman, New York).

Ethical Principles

transmogrification of subject into object, of man into a thing, against which the destructive urge may wreak its fury without restraint.

The same sentiment was forcibly echoed by Dr. Bean,[1]

The degradation of physicians in Germany exemplifies the decline and fall of a group whose moral obligations went by default in a single generation. The house would not have fallen had not many of the timbers been rotten. Descent into the gas chambers by doctors of infamy had its beginings in disregard for patients. The patient, however humble, and however ill, in whatever degree derelict and forlorn, has sacred rights which the physician must always put ahead of his burning curiosity.

A recent issue of *Saturday Review* contains the following report from an American psychologist:[2]

But this group of data-happy physicians have company in every behavioral science. Several years ago one of our undergraduates spent the summer in another university as a research assistant. Her 'responsibility' was to entice college freshmen into cheating on tests while social psychologists used one-way mirrors and listening devices to study the freshmen's cheating and consequent breakdown when confronted with *their* immoral behaviour. A scientist at Harvard enjoys telling his professional audiences that the cruelty exhibited in the Nazi concentration camps is latent in many Americans. He has proved this by forcing subjects to administer what they believe to be dangerous electric shocks to other subjects (accomplices of the experimenter) who beg not to be tortured further and who scream pitifully when they receive the shocks. He has, I think, unwittingly assumed the role of the concentration camp doctor.

All these studies were made without the subjects, usually college students, knowing in advance that they might be subjected to stress. As a matter of fact most subjects had to participate in these and other studies in order to fulfil requirements for a course in general psychology.

[1] W. B. Bean, of Iowa, *Journal of Laboratory and Clinical Medicine*, 1952, **39**, 3.
[2] R. H. Bixler, of University of Louisville, Kentucky, in *Saturday Review* (page 47), 2 July 1966.

Principles

Proposed codes concerning human experimentation

The best-known ethical code governing doctor-patient relationships is that of Hippocrates (460–370 B.C.), who expressed the view that the profession of medicine could not survive without a sound moral philosophy, and formulated his famous oath. But, whereas thirty years ago a large percentage of British and American medical schools insisted that all doctors take this oath on graduation, this procedure occurs in very few medical schools today, and, in the vast majority, nothing has been substituted. Undoubtedly many of the clauses of the Hippocratic oath are unacceptable today.

The so-called Nuremberg Code is a judicial summary of the expert testimony presented in the case against the Nazi doctors accused of war crimes. It is important to understand that the judgement rendered by the Nuremberg Military Tribunal concerning human experimentation has never been and probably never will be construed either in Britain or America as legal precedent. The code consists of ten clauses of which the first is the most important and is developed in the greatest detail compared with the others. It deserves to be quoted in full:[1]

> The voluntary consent of the human subject is absolutely essential. This means that the person involved should have legal capacity to give consent; should be so situated as to be able to exercise free power of choice, without the intervention of any element of force, fraud, deceit, duress, over-reaching, or other ulterior form of constraint or coercion; and should have sufficient knowledge and comprehension of the elements of the subject matter involved as to enable him to make an understanding and enlightened decision. The latter element requires that before the acceptance of an affirmative decision by the experimental subject there should be made known to him the nature, duration, and purpose of the experiment; the method and means by which it is to be conducted; all inconveniences and hazards reasonably to be expected; and the effects upon his health or person which may possibly come from his participation in the experiment. The duty and responsibility for ascertaining the quality of the consent rests upon each individual who initiates, directs, or engages in the experiment. It is a personal duty and responsibility which may not be delegated to another with impunity."

[1] Quoted in *Journal American Medical Association*, 1946, **132,** 1090.

Ethical Principles

The House of Delegates of the American Medical Association adopted the report of their Judicial Council on requirements for human experimentation which formulated the following three principles:[1]

1. The voluntary consent of the person on whom the experiment is to be performed must be obtained.
2. The danger of each experiment must have been investigated previously by means of animal experimentation.
3. The experiment must be performed under proper medical protection and management.

The World Medical Association formulated a set of rules concerning human experimentation in 1955,[2] which were rewritten in 1961[3] and again very recently.[4]

My own suggested headings for a code concerning human experimentation would be concerned with the following principles: equality; valid consent; prohibited subjects; previous animal experiments; experimenters' competence; proper records. Some comments about each of these principles will be given.

I. The principle of equality

No experiment should be contemplated, proposed or undertaken to which, if he were in circumstances identical to those of the intended subjects, the experimenter would even hesitate to submit himself, or members of his own family, or anybody for whom he had any respect or affection. This principle of equality should be the corner-stone of the whole edifice of any code. It is essentially a restatement of the Golden Rule preached by Jesus and the advice given by Rabbi Hillel a hundred years earlier, 'Do not unto any man that which you would not have done to yourself.'

In a personal letter to me, dated 6 April 1966, Professor Ivy of Roosevelt University, Chicago, Illinois, wrote:

> The principle of The Golden Rule and that the means should not in time negate a good end, are basic principles. Furthermore, the idea that the experimenter is worth more than the

[1] *Journal American Medical Association*, 1946, **132**, 1090.
[2] *World Medical Journal*, 1955, **2**, 14.
[3] *British Medical Journal*, 1962, **2**, 1119.
[4] *Clinical Research* (Washington), 1966, **14**, 193.

subject is ruinous. This ideology has crept into American clinical investigation to some extent. In 1947 I predicted that it would do so. The Nazis thought that they were the best people on earth and could do no wrong when working either for the good of the state or for the good of Society. The feeling of superiority has ruined civilizations, nations, groups and individuals.

What experimenter, hoping for whatever results for research, would submit his own child, aged less than twelve months, and free from heart trouble, to cardiac catheterization (page 35)? What experimenter would be happy that his own wife, pregnant and suffering no abnormality, should be subjected, in the interests of science, to translumbar aortography (page 48)? And what experimenter, considering whatever advance might be made in research by his results, would agree to the subjection of one of his parents, who was fatally ill, to the development of a technique such as retrograde arterial catheterization (pages 71, 155) in order that the experimenters may learn that particular technique? How comforted would he feel, after learning that a serious and painful complication had, in this case, resulted from the experiment, to learn from the experimenters' report that the number of such complications, while considerable, is regarded by them as 'not prohibitively high' and that 'New techniques encounter difficulties until they are perfected'?

If no experimenter would act in these ways towards someone close to him, surely it is wrong for him to do so towards someone he doesn't know – and is never going to know – 'a case'. For this reason I have called this principle, from which the other five principles follow, the principle of equality.

Moreover, the number involved in any experiment is from an ethical point of view completely immaterial. If it is unethical for one, it is for the many. The reverse is also true, namely, if it is unethical to submit many to a proposed experiment, it is equally unethical to expose only one person.

2. *The principle of valid consent*

The importance of valid consent is emphasized in all codes of principles for human research. I am in full agreement with all the details concerning consent listed in the Nuremberg Code, which has been quoted fully previously.

The Medical Research Council of Britain in 1953 issued a memorandum on human experimentation, and regarding consent made the following apposite, if perhaps inconclusive, remarks:[1]

> But familiarity (of the physician) with novelty should not lead us to forget that, to the patient, every procedure which lies outside his idea of the expected routine of medical care, is still likely to cause apprehension and may lead to misunderstanding or even mistrust unless the justification for its use in his case has been made amply clear to him.
>
> To obtain the consent of the patient to a proposed investigation is not in itself enough. Owing to the special relationship of trust which exists between a patient and his doctor, most patients will consent to any proposals that are made. Further, the considerations involved are so technical as to prevent their being adequately understood by one who is not himself an expert.

Two essential pieces of information are often deliberately withheld from 'the consenting volunteer', namely, that the procedure is experimental and its consequences are unpredictable.

> The medical research procedure by definition and by nature is a deviation from normal practice, even though all the specific elements involved may be well established, simply because medical practice ordinarily does not encompass employment of human beings primarily for advancement of knowledge. There is no implicit understanding that conventional methods will be used and that the patient will be released as soon as his condition warrants. Consequently, the researcher has a more specific responsibility for full disclosure of purpose, method and probable consequences.[2]

The fact that consent is often not only not asked but that it is often *deliberately* not asked has been pointed out by Professor McCance, who asserted, in 1951, that in some European

[1] Medical Research Council *Memorandum* 649, issued 16 October 1953.

[2] Irving Ladimer, S.J.D. of Law-Medicine Institute, Boston University, *Journal of Public Law*, 1955, **3**, 467.

medical centres 'the co-operation of patient or parent is seldom sought, and in some places it is generally assumed that it would be refused'.[1] That this should be so merely underlines the vital importance of consent. For if the consent, when asked, is likely to be refused, it will only be refused because of the personal wishes and fears of the patient. In keeping the subject in the dark as to what is being done to him so as to avoid a refusal, the experimenter is, in fact, guilty of a fraud. Indeed, a very distinguished Guy's surgeon, Sir William Ogilvie, whom I have already quoted[2] and in the same article, has said exactly this.

> What is new in medicine is research by fraud. The performance on patients, who have come to us in good faith for the cure of their ailments, of any number of tests and investigations, many of them unnecessary for the diagnosis or treatment of their ailments, but are performed in a general search for information, or merely as a bit of practice in technique.[3]

Dr. Cullinan of St. Bartholomew's Hospital, London, put the matter very plainly at a meeting of the Royal Society of Medicine, London, when he expressed the opinion:

> Sticking needles and catheters into patients in guise of treatment, when what was done was really in search of knowledge, seems very near to common assault.[4]

A lawyer has stated the case equally strongly:

> One of the major malpractices of our era consists in the engineering of consent. Sometimes this is effected by simply exploiting the condition of necessitous men. . . . Then again, consent may be engineered by the kind of psychologist who takes it for granted that his assistants and students will submit to experiments and implies a threat to advancement if they raise objections. Or the total community may engineer a consent, as when the president, the generals, and the newspapers call with loud fanfare for a heroic crew of astronautical volunteers to attempt some ultrahazardous exploit.[5]

[1] *Proceedings of the Royal Society of Medicine*, 1951, **44**, 189.
[2] Page 8 of this book.
[3] *Lancet*, 1952, **2**, 820.
[4] *Lancet*, 1958, **1**, 944.
[5] E. Cahn, Professor of Law, New York University, *New York Law Review*, 1961, **36**, 1.

Ethical Principles

In many cases where apparently consent is asked and obtained there is so little candour toward the subject that, although in the event consent is given, the subject really has no proper idea of what he has consented to. The following instance will illustrate what I mean. Some time ago I was talking to a well-known London cardiologist in the presence of three other doctors. I asked his opinion about a series of unpublished experiments which had come to my notice in which dental patients, who were having teeth extracted under anaesthesis, also underwent, without knowing it, cardiac catherization while under the anaesthetic. By this means samples of blood were in each case taken direct from the heart. Our conversation went like this:

> Myself: 'Do you consider this to have been a reasonable and justifiable experiment?'
> Cardiologist: 'Yes.'
> Myself: 'Would you not first have asked the patient's permission?'
> Cardiologist: 'Yes.'
> Myself: 'What would you have told them?'
> Cardiologist: 'I would have explained that we were going to obtain a few small blood samples for examination to see if organisms got into the blood stream immediately after dental extraction.'
> Myself: 'Would you tell them how you intended to obtain the blood?'
> Cardiologist: 'No, it would be quite unnecessary to do so.'
> Myself: 'Would you regard this as constituting valid consent?'
> Cardiologist: 'Definitely, yes.'
> Myself: 'Don't you think there would be an element of fraud in this?'
> Cardiologist: 'Certainly not.'

With regard to the age of consent, an English lawyer, who is also a doctor, has written:[1]

> The age at which consent to treatment may be accepted as valid has never been settled in the English courts. Age of attainment of legal capacity varies for different purposes – for example, a person under 21 years cannot make a valid will

[1] Gavin Thurston, who is Her Majesty's Coroner for Inner West London *British Medical Journal*, 1966, **1**, 1405.

or vote at an election or enter into a binding contract. On the other hand, young persons can marry at 16; a girl of 16 may consent to sexual intercourse without the risk of criminal proceedings against her partner; and The Children and Young Persons Acts cease to apply at 17.

The vast majority of published accounts of experiments on patients, including most of the reports quoted in this book, do not mention whether or not consent has been asked or obtained. This omission does not entitle us automatically to assume that consent was not sought or not obtained. We just do not know.

This ambiguity may cause injustice to experimenters who have obtained genuine valid consent. The fault lies with the writers themselves and the editors of medical articles, who should always not only state but give unequivocal evidence of having obtained genuine and legally valid consent.

3. *The principle of prohibited subjects*

Experiments should under no circumstances be performed on mentally sick patients, whatever may be the technical designation of their particular mental illness. Nor should experiments ever be performed on the aged or the dying.

Many doctors, including some in high places, would object to these prohibitions, seeing nothing wrong in such procedures. But they must be indefensible if we take the principle of equality and valid consent seriously. Someone whose mental capacity is impaired, whether permanently or temporarily, cannot be expected to understand properly the purpose and means of an experiment, even if, as is hardly ever the case with this group of subjects, any attempt is made to explain them. The use of such subjects is, in fact, little more than a quick and easy way of obtaining 'experimental material' without considering consent at all.

Should prison inmates be included within this category of prohibited subjects? In Britain, where such subjects are never used, the question does not arise. There are those, however, as was noted in the section dealing with this practice, who advocate that the system should be adopted in Britain. Perhaps a case could be made out for the use of prison inmates, provided there was valid consent and proper terms of compensation were included in a contract. But I think that the following consideration rules this out. If the experiment is quite innocuous, then the offer of a reward for those who undergo it is unfair to those who have not had the chance to participate. If, however, the experiment is not innocuous, as has been the case with some conducted in American prisons, and this was probably the reason why these men were approached in the first place, then the procedure deserves condemnation. To subject prison inmates to procedures which may injure them is a cheap trick played on men who are taking their punishment. Prison inmates, then, are a group on whom no experiments should be performed.

Many patients in hospitals, besides being ill with a physical ailment, are emotionally disturbed, either because of that particular sickness or just because they are ill. These patients will be in a 'nervous' condition and it is the obvious duty of those in whose care they are to avoid anything which is likely to increase the patient's anxiety. An experiment, especially an experiment of some of the kinds that have been described in this book, is likely to worry such a patient more than others and the question of consent in such cases may also be more difficult to meet properly. Obviously nervous or psychically disturbed patients should, for these reasons, be automatically excluded from all experiments. It is clear, I think, that the same reasoning should be applied to the aged, who, in fact, are more likely to be nervous than other patients and who are probably less able to grasp an explanation and more afraid of saying no.

The use of patients who are dying as subjects for experiments is shocking and wrong. This should hardly need saying. Indeed, in the case of the dying, the doctors should perhaps be hesitant even about the use of an untried therapeutic technique, even though the patient may agree, especially if he is afraid of dying, as he may agree to anything. I myself have seen the trial use of new agents in cancer where the suffering produced by the agent in question has been very much worse than the suffering caused by the disease itself. Where a patient cannot be saved, it is common humanity that he should be allowed to die in peace.

Principles

Some experimenters have allowed themselves to believe, where the subject of their proposed experiment is a patient with an incurable disease, that a risky experiment is for that reason justified. Quite apart from the unpleasantness of the experiment itself, and quite apart from the risk of worsening the patient's condition if things go wrong, there is the question of what is meant by 'incurable'. As Dr. Guttentag has pointed out,

> From the experimenter's point of view the description 'hopelessly incurable' is not germane to his purpose. The designation is inadequate, because it does not specify the time-element – hopeless within hours, days, months, years? And if months or years are concerned, do all experts agree on the status of their respective sciences and deny the possibility of discovering effective agents within such a period? From the standpoint of the physician-friend their assertion is not germane to his purpose either. To him it is an expression of detachment between physician and patient, the announcement of a scale of partnership, viz, domination, quite contrary to its original spirit. As a matter of fact it creates the paradox that the healthier the patient the more he should be the concern of the physician; the sicker, the less.[1]

By avoiding altogether experiments on the incurable the doctors would secure themselves against the anomalous moral positions which Guttentag here indicates. Indeed, many experimenters seem to consider that the labelling of a patient as 'hopeless' or 'incurable' gives them permission for greater boldness than would be used in dealing with other patients.

4. *The principle of previous animal experimentation*

In nearly every suggested code for experiments this has been recommended; and it is only comparatively rarely that animal experiments are not possible before human ones. Lack of laboratory facilities should never be an excuse for not using animals first since any experimenter who lacks such facilities should not be doing experiments at all. An exception to the prior use of animals is the case of research into mental disease where the analogous condition does not exist in animals. Here the problems are special. The use of mental patients as controls

[1] O. E. Guttentag, of University of California Medical School, *Science*, 1953, **117,** 207.

for experiments unconnected with their own condition should be ruled out in any case, as I have already said. In far too many instances, however, the simple rule of experimenting first on animals is disregarded. Human experiments are less trouble and, as I shall mention later, at present no form-filling nor any record-keeping is necessary before a human experiment is undertaken; with animals both are necessary.

Some reasons why animal experiments are often by-passed are mentioned in a recent article which points out that, in contrast to an animal which must by law nearly always be anaesthetized before an experiment, a human subject very often need not be.[1] This gives the experimenter two advantages. First, a man can be 'awake and responsive throughout the study'. Second, 'the investigator need not be concerned about the influence of an anaesthetic agent'.

The same article continues:

> But certainly whenever feasible the investigator will choose man as his subject rather than a laboratory animal. As obvious as this may appear, many clinical investigators spend a great deal of time and effort using expensive equipment in studies on laboratory animals, when the same studies could be conducted safely on man. . . . The clinical investigator must never forget that the 'proper study of mankind is man'. More research is needed on the greatest of all animals – man.

The keyword of this quotation is, of course, 'safely'. One fears that the view presented by the authors, and which is that held by many experimenters, is that having to work with animals first is something not strictly necessary or useful. In fact, prior animal experiments are of great use, of which a very important part is that by means of them many risky, unpleasant and futile experiments on human subjects can be avoided altogether.

In England there appears to be more concern for the welfare of animals than for sick patients. It is interesting to note, as recorded by the distinguished physician who was an important medical witness for the prosecution at the Nuremberg trial, that Hitler when he first assumed power issued an edict making all

[1] G. E. Burch and De Pasquale, of Tulane University, New Orleans, *American Heart Journal*, 1964, **67**, 287.

animal experiments illegal. But this he followed up by ordering the mass murder of inmates of mental hospitals.[1]

Another example which illustrates the care taken in England to safeguard animals is that Her Majesty's Stationery Office publishes each year a very detailed account of vivisection experiments and this is open to the scrutiny of anybody who cares to buy a copy. I seriously advocate that a similar list be published of all experiments done on hospital patients, giving full details of the nature and purpose of each experiment.

5. *The principle of the experimenter's competence*

Many of those who take part in experiments are not themselves qualified in medicine, although during an experiment they are working under medical supervision. It is very important that, in such cases, the parts played by people who are actually unqualified medically should be limited to what they can do with complete safety. As Professor McCance has written,

> Many experimental workers (e.g. laboratory technicians) are not qualified in medicine and yet they take part (under medical supervision) in hospital work and experiments on 'normal' people. Could they conceivably be regarded as 'unqualified assistants' and what would be the position if an accident were found to be due to one of them?[2]

There is at present a clamour for research facilities to be extended so that physicians in outlying hospitals can enter this field. If these facilities are to be provided it is very important that the patients who may become the subjects of experiments undertaken in hospitals which so far do not go in for research should be safeguarded by the responsibility for experiments being shared by a number of senior staff. If an experiment is conceived, carried out and answered for by a single physician, there may well be too little protection of the interests of those on whom it is performed. Experiments on human beings should never be undertaken by the lone investigator.

6. *The principle of proper records*

The reasons why proper records should be kept by the experimenters and *included in the patient's records* are obvious, though

[1] Professor Ivy, of Chicago, *Journal American Medical Association*, 1949, **139**, 131.
[2] *Proceedings Royal Society Medicine*, 1951, **44**, 189.

often disregarded. Simply, if a patient consents to be the subject of an experiment and then undergoes that experiment, what has been done to him is virtually part of his medical history. This is so in any case and it applies particularly if any unexpected reaction or any complication occurs. Quite often, when a complication does occur, repeated or different side-effects can appear much later. And if the patient's records contain no account of this, then the doctor who attends the patient at a later date will not be getting the full story. Neglect of proper records is thus against the interests of the patient himself, against those of his doctors and against the interests of medicine.

Furthermore, I advocate legislation to make it compulsory for all doctors to report all deaths and major complications directly and indirectly due to any experimental investigation to a central bureau at the Ministry of Health, and that severe penalties be instituted for ignoring this order.

Objection to ethical codes

In general most doctors favour the formulation and acceptance of some code as a guidance concerning human experimentation. For example, this is the view strongly expressed in an editorial in the *New England Journal of Medicine* (1960, **262**, 1090). But some doctors have been but mildly lukewarm in their acceptance of any suggested code. A recent editorial states:[1]

> It seems that the best safeguard of the public interest lies not in exhaustive codes of ethics but rather in the ethical consensus of clinical investigators as reflected in peer judgement.

Criticism of the suggested codes may be briefly summarized as follows:

1. They are not enforceable.
2. They have no legal sanction.
3. There is frequent disagreement and quibbling concerning specific parts of every suggested code and each critic wishes to alter some clause to make it conform to his own viewpoint, and possibly thereby make it evident that the code does not condemn in any way his own research activities.

[1] *Clinical Research* (Washington), 1966, **14**, 193.

4. Some doctors even dispute the need for any ethical code.
5. Some complain that they are unduly restrictive, hampering medical progress.
6. The abysmal (possibly sometimes purposeful) ambiguity of the wording of part of some codes. For example, clause 3 of the code prepared in 1963 by the Ethical Committee of the British Medical Association states:

> No new technique or investigation should be undertaken on any patient unless it is strictly necessary for the treatment of the patient.

But how can anybody prove that any new technique, especially if previously untried, is strictly necessary for the treatment of a particular patient?

Another example is clause 3 of the World Medical Association code:

> Clinical research cannot legitimately be carried out unless the importance of the objective is in proportion to the inherent risk to the subject.

I feel confident that many research workers whose experiments are summarized in this volume would contend that their own work was in conformity with this precept, but I, for one, would dispute this. Moreover, several clauses of this code contain the phrase 'of benefit to the subject or others', a concept which, for reasons previously stated, I find wholly unacceptable.

Undoubtedly no code can ever be a substitute for the moral integrity of any individual investigator. No code will curb the unscrupulous. No appeal to the conscience will be effective with anybody who lacks a conscience. For these reasons and after careful thought over many years I have reluctantly come to the conclusion that the voluntary system of safeguarding patients' rights has failed and new legislative procedures are absolutely necessary.

2. LEGAL CONSIDERATIONS

Four recent quotations from American sources are of considerable interest and relevance:

> Human experimentation is as ancient as the practice of medicine, yet, remarkably enough, no specified legal prece-

dents have been set down to protect the subject or the investigator. At the same time there is abundance of precedent to indicate that however able, skilful, conscientious, well trained and generally well qualified the investigator is, he experiments on man to his peril.[1]

The law is difficult to interpret because, although it is technically inaccurate to state that 'there is no law' on the subject of human experimentation, it is true that there are no statutes and no reported cases dealing directly with clinical investigation as such. However, medical research activity, like all activities in our society, is subject to common-law principles of general applicability. Since neither the legislatures nor the courts have found it necessary to determine the specific application of these general principles to clinical research, the 'law' governing this activity remains, within certain well-defined limits, somewhat uncertain, or, more precisely, undeveloped.[2]

Physicians and medical scientists who find it necessary to test hypotheses by exposing human beings to unestablished procedures, generally declare that they follow the primary Hippocratic tenet, prescribing that they should do no harm. There has, however, not yet crystallized a set of specific guidelines, commonly understood and applicable, to insure that human research may go forward on the highest scientific and ethical planes with due legal protection for both the subject and the investigator. . . .

Taking a leaf from the book of strictures governing malpractice, it is clear that malpractice connotes any conduct on the part of the physician not in line with good or standard medical practice. The physician's failure to meet the standard may be due to (1) ignorance or lack of skill, (2) wilful departure from accepted practice, (3) negligence, (4) breach of positive law, such as failure to obtain consent. Malpractice applies equally for these reasons to the research scientist who fails to meet the controlling standards or guides governing the profession of scientific investigation. These are more subtle and more difficult, since the essence of research is novel and untried activity, but the means by which research is planned or undertaken and the safeguards employed are essentially similar, even

[1] H. K. Beecher, of Harvard Medical School, *Journal American Medical Association*, 1959, **169**, 461.
[2] *Clinical Investigation*, Legal, Ethical and Moral Aspects, page 169 (Boston University Research Institute, 1963).

though – as in medical practice – the particular diagnosis, observation, or treatment is unique.[1]

An offensive touching or invasion of the body, if not consented to, is a trespass against the person, a battery redressible in an action for damages. Even the consent of the victim is no defence to a charge of homicide. . . . If a human life is deliberately taken it is, moreover, no mitigation of the crime that the victim was by worldly standards someone of little merit, or someone having little time left to live. The governing standard is not the merit or need or value of the victim but the equality of worth as a human being. . . . Even the saving of lives will not justify the taking of a life.[2]

In Britain the legal validity of human experimentation has never been tested in law. In an annual report the Medical Defence Society of Britain commented:

We were asked on more than one occasion to advise on the legal aspects of research and experimentation in medicine. . . . The real difficulty arises in regard to persons who are ill. We have been asked whether a form of consent signed by the patient could effectively protect the doctors. We have advised that a signed form of consent might assist, but it would be most unwise for a doctor to rely entirely on it.

The British legal view has been stated by Dr. Mackintosh, who emphasized that valid consent is essential and added:

The law in England is by no means clear as to the responsibility of the experimenter in the case of accident arising. The maxim 'volente non fit injuris', still holds, and might be freely expressed as, 'volunteers cannot claim damages'. . . . Whether co-operation in the event of accident is covered by consent in writing of the patient is a matter which would have to be tested in the court.[3]

To me it appears obvious from these quotations that some legislation is needed for the responsible and conscientious experimenter. As the law stands he may, in the case of an accident, be liable to prosecution for assault or trespass.

[1] I. Ladimer, S.J.D., *Journal of Public Law*, 1955, **3**, 467.
[2] Professor F. A. Freund, *New England Journal of Medicine*, 1965, **273**, 687.
[3] J. M. Mackintosh, who is a British doctor acting as consultant to the United States Public Health Service. Quoted by Beecher, *Journal American Medical Association*, 1959, **169**, 461.

Legal Considerations

By far the most important reason, however, why there should be legislation on this matter is the need to protect the public. This reason has been consistently treated as insufficient, and the need for changes in the law denied, by successive Ministers of Health. Thus Mr. Macleod, the then Minister of Health, when questioned in the House of Commons in 1955 about an experiment with penicillin that had been carried out in Bristol, replied that:

> Only the clinician in charge could say what was right and proper and what safeguards were needed in the action he took . . . He thought it would be entirely improper for him to try to lay down what ethical and moral principles should govern the conduct of professional men in the work they undertook in hospitals. . . . He is absolutely convinced that it would be quite wrong for a Minister of Health to issue directions on a matter that is essentially one of medical ethics, to those concerned. He was sure that it was best to leave the matter to the profession, and not to have a lay Minister interfering in a matter that was very precious to those professionally concerned . . . Of one thing he was clear: no direction must come from the Minister on a matter of this delicacy.

Three years later Mr. Walker-Smith (Minister of Health in that year) in answer to another question in the House of Commons – this time concerning experiments on mental defectives – took the same line and replied simply that, 'investigations of this kind involve medical and ethical problems which are not susceptible to control by legislation'.

A third instance of 'passing-by-on-the-side' occurred in 1962. In October of that year two Members of Parliament asked the Minister (Mr. Powell) under what conditions experiments were permitted and to what extent they were carried out without consent. (These questions arose from the publication of my article in *Twentieth Century* on the subject.) In his reply Mr. Powell informed the House that guidance on this subject had been given to all hospital authorities in a letter dated January 1959 and added: 'I have no reason to suppose that that guidance is not generally observed.'

The argument against legislation by these successive Ministers, then boils down to the contentions that: (*a*) it is unnecessary because nothing is wrong, and (*b*) that even if something were wrong the subject is 'essentially one of medical ethics' and that a lay Minister should not interfere in 'a matter that was very precious to those professionally concerned'. The first of these contentions does not, I feel, require further refutation. The second is easily shown as an evasion of the real issue if we remember two things. The first is that the people who require protection are not those who are 'professionally concerned' and to whom the matter may be 'very precious', who themselves are in no danger whatever of pain, injury or the indignity of being made experimental subjects without their free consent. The people who require protection are lay people who are, or may be, at present exposed to these dangers and to this indignity. The second is that, on related issues, which could equally easily be relegated to the conscience and sole trust of those 'professionally concerned', and which are equally questions of ethics, our laws do not place the entire authority to decide what is permissible and what is not in the hands of a professional class. Ironically, experiments on animals, which are, of course, conducted by doctors engaged in research, are strictly controlled by Act of Parliament. Before such experiments can be carried out licences must be obtained, and to obtain them the experimenters must state in detail the purpose and nature of what they are proposing to do. Animal experiments are not simply regarded as a matter which is 'essentially one of medical ethics' and about which, therefore, no law need stand on the Statute Book. Indeed, not only are licences required by law before animal experiments are undertaken, but as recently as 1962 the Government agreed to appoint additional inspectors to ensure that the law in this matter was properly observed.[1]

A special Act of Parliament had to be passed recently so that surgeons could, legally, remove the cornea (for subsequent grafting) from the body of a person who had 'bequeathed his eyes'. And even with this law, and where the eyes have been bequeathed, it remains legally necessary for permission to be granted by the person's relative before the corneas may be removed.

It is possible to trace, over the past fifty years, a gradual

[1] As recommended by a Cruelty to Animals Advisory Committee set up by the Government under the chairmanship of Lord Morris of Borth-y-Gest.

improvement in the status of patients. This is something entirely good, although there still remains in just this area room
for much more improvement. Thus before 1914 surgeons in
Great Britain very rarely bothered to obtain written, or even
verbal, consent to the operations which they performed. It was
assumed that hospital patients automatically accepted without
demur or question any treatment, medical or surgical, which
was given them. This attitude stemmed largely from the
general attitude doctors maintained toward what they called
'the hospital class', the view that such patients were in general
of inferior intelligence, less sensitive than others and altogether
of not very great importance. In some parts of the U.S.A. this
attitude to non-fee-paying, uninsured 'charity patients' still
seems to exist. But in Britain, after the introduction of the
National Insurance Scheme in 1914 and of the National Health
Service in 1948 patients have been gradually learning to know
and on occasions even to demand their rights.

It has been the accepted practice in Britain since about
1914 for a nurse to obtain written consent from the patient or
(in the case of a child) from a parent or guardian, prior to any
operation, though not prior to an investigation. A very important question about patients entering hospital is whether
they are *bound*, by doing so, to submit to any investigation or
treatment ordered by the doctor in whose care they are or
whether, and to what extent, they may question or decline such
treatment. Before 1939 I have myself seen on several occasions
patients ordered to be discharged immediately from hospital
for daring to question the treatment meted out to them. It is to
be feared that this unequal and presumptuous attitude still
sometimes prevails.

The position in this matter is still somewhat equivocal and
the question of what constitutes consent is not always quite
clear. An example of this occurred in 1954, when a woman
patient wrote to the Management Committee of the Royal
Hospital, Wolverhampton, complaining that an operation had
been performed on her ear without consent. The secretary of
the committee replied:

> It is not in order for surgical treatment to be given without the
> patient's consent, but consent can be implied when a patient
> comes into hospital for examination. If a patient comes to

hospital, either on his doctor's advice or his own initiative, he is deemed to agree to receive treatment.[1]

From a legal point of view this is almost certainly a bad ruling. Recently an authoritative opinion has been expressed,

> The nature of the operation must be explained by a medical practitioner and not by a nurse. Unless a proper explanation has been given the mind of the patient cannot go with the signature, and the so-called 'consent' does not exist. This is why the doctor must countersign the certificate and add the date. The practice of having the patient sign a blank consent form on reception into hospital cannot be too strongly deprecated.[2]

If, with regard to experiments on animals, doctors are bound by law, and if it is the accepted practice and acknowledged as right that a patient's consent must be obtained before any operation is performed, even though it is directly aimed at treating his disease, then doctors should surely be equally bound in the matter of human experimentation. Surely the only objection to such laws (provided they embodied the principles outlined previously) would be from those who wished to ignore these principles, and not from those who wish to abide by them. Legislation is needed and would be no impediment to the conscientious experimenter who already conforms to what such law would make compulsory.

As far as I am aware there have been no cases in Britain within recent years of any patient having been awarded damages in a court of law in a claim against an experimental physician. However, such actions may have been started but settled out of court, and so have never come to light. Moreover, in any such legal action it would be very difficult to persuade any expert medical witness to give evidence on behalf of a patient-plaintiff.

There is a further reason for seriously advocating legislation in respect of medical experiments – the financial aspect. Such experiments cost money and, since a not inconsiderable proportion of this money comes from the taxpayer, it seems right that, through the laws of this country, he should have a say in

---

[1] Quoted in *Lancet*, 1954, **1**, 421.

[2] Gavin Thurston, who is a doctor and lawyer, *British Medical Journal*, 1966, **1**, 1405.

the way that this part of his money is spent.[1] Much of the money required for medical research does, it is true, come from private sources which include, besides individual benefactors, industrial concerns and, in particular, pharmaceutical manufacturers. But it also comes in Britain from three public sources: the National Health Service, University Grants, and the Medical Research Council. Research workers in Britain often complain about the smallness of the contribution toward the cost of their work made by the National Health Service. But what is often overlooked is that the cost of keeping patients in hospital (that is, of providing the greater number of the subjects for their experiments) is born entirely by the National Health Service, that much of the laboratory equipment (true, sometimes the least expensive) is bought out of National Health Service funds, and that they themselves draw a substantial part of their income from the same source. Directly or indirectly, in Britain a big part of the bill for medical experiments is paid by the Government, who thus should be responsible for the prevention of abuses and entitled to enact laws accordingly. At the same time it would be well if private benefactors and trustees acting for them were better enlightened as to the precise means for which their donations were often used.

Some figures will give an idea of the amount of money spent on medical research in America. In 1945 the Massachusetts General Hospital had available for research 500,000 dollars per year. In 1965 this had risen to 8,384,342 dollars, which is a remarkable seventeenfold increase in twenty years. The National Institute of Health increase during the same period has been a gigantic 624-fold, from 700,000 dollars annually to 437,000,000 dollars. And all this represents only a small fraction of the total spent in America on medical research. Another index is that the National Institute of Health awarded over 500 postgraduate research fellowships annually. In addition there are the voluntary organizations who donate huge sums for special research such as cancer, poliomyelitis, multiple sclerosis and heart disease, through their 'fellowship programs'. In 1961 the Federal Government grant for medical research was 904

[1] The *British Medical Journal* for 4 July 1964 quotes the figures given in the House on 17 June 1964 of what H.M. Government has in recent years spent on medical research. In the financial year 1962/3 this amount was £16 million.

million dollars, which was three times that of 1956. The dona-
tion of the American Heart Association in 1965 was 32,500,000
dollars. The estimated amount spent on heart research alone in
America in 1963 was nearly 200,000,000 dollars.

3. PROPOSED LEGISLATION

If it is accepted that there is a definite case for Parliamentary or
Federal legislation to control human experimentation, then it
seems clear that what is needed is an Act or Statute. Such an
Act, embodying the ethical principles set out previously, could
function through some existing authority or one created by the
new Act. Let us consider the question of this authority.

A practising physician who is also an experimental investigator is not qualified to judge objectively if the risks involved in
any experiments on his own patients are justifiable. His necessarily objective 'scientific' attitude is likely, at least occasionally
if not frequently, to conflict with that of a true doctor-patient
relationship.

> The physician-experimenter is liable to be an eager, obsessional
> fellow who may overbear the physician-friend; when they are
> united in the same body, the patient may suffer.[1]

So, whether or not any proposed experiment is legally and
ethically justifiable must never be the sole opinion and decision
of the experimenter himself or his team, but must always be the
decision of properly constituted consultation committees. Each
large hospital or, preferably, hospital group must have a committee of doctors, but one member must be a clinician who
himself is not engaged in any research, and there should be at
least one lay member, preferably but not necessarily a lawyer.
In Britain each Regional Hospital Board would have such a
committee, but the independence of the teaching hospitals of
these Boards may be a difficult procedural point.

In Britain each research committee should be responsible to
the General Medical Council, whose own authority in the
matter would be accordingly extended. The General Medical
Council in its turn would be answerable to Parliament. The
use of the existing machinery is suggested because when the

---

[1] Gavin Thurston, of London, *British Medical Journal*, 1966, **1**, 1405.

Proposed Legislation

General Medical Council was set up by Act of Parliament the legislative intention was the creation of an official body whose main purpose should be to protect the lay public. As Sir David Campbell, a recent President of the General Medical Council, has said,

> The declared purpose of Parliament was not to promote the welfare of professional men nor of professional corporations, such as the Royal Colleges; it was not to put down quackery or even to advance medical science. The object was simply the interest and protection of the public.[1]

If this were followed, then it would be a function of the General Medical Council to receive and investigate any complaints made to it direct by members of the public, as well as to supervise generally the implementation of the provisions of the Act by the research committees.

Each research committee, besides being responsible for deciding on whether an experiment could be undertaken or not, would, in the case of those which it did sanction, receive a full report from the doctors who have conducted it. This report should include the following information:

1. Aim of experiment.
2. Age, medical and mental condition of all subjects before the experiment.
3. Evidence of free and comprehending consent. In the case of a non-patient volunteer evidence that there was no coercion and of group and not individual approach. Evidence, in all cases, that consent was obtained by the doctor in charge of the experiment and that the asking of consent was not delegated.
4. History of experiment. Including an account of any distress, pain, injury or accident occurring to the subject.
5. Time occupied.
6. Confirmation that all necessary safeguards were taken.
7. Post-experimental condition of the subject and mention of all and every complication, even if considered minor.
8. Confirmation that, in the case of a patient, a copy of this record has been included in the patient's notes.

[1] *British Medical Journal*, 1962, **2**, 561.

9. Confirmation that in the case of death resulting directly or indirectly from any experiment the coroner has been informed.

On this last point the position in Britain is needlessly obscured by the fact that although doctors are under statutary obligation to report such deaths to the coroner this rule is frequently ignored. Yet I know of no instance where such infringement has led to legal action against the doctor concerned. In Canada there is a Coroner's Act with strict enforcement of the rule that if any patient dies directly or indirectly as a result of any treatment given to him in hospital then the death and its circumstances must be reported to the coroner on pain of severe penalties. Defaulters can also be summoned for a breach of the Vital Statistics Act. In 1954 five doctors were in trouble for not reporting such fatalities.[1]

The Medical Research Committees' reports, whether the individual experiments have been published in medical journals or not, should be sent to a central registry office, which should annually publish a brief summary of all human experiments undertaken, as is now done in Britain for animal experiments.

A further innovation which would be of great help in restoring morality to research could be made, without any legislation, by medical editors. At the present time it is often considered essential, for the young doctor intent on promotion, to be able to point to the publication of his own articles in medical journals. Such publication undoubtedly increases the chances of advancement and there is little doubt that the motive behind a certain amount of medical writing, and also behind the research which is very often the subject of such writing, is more the personal ambition of the doctor than his real desire to help medicine itself. To object to this may be regarded as over-idealistic, and perhaps it would be, but for one thing. Many of the experiments which form the subject-matter of such articles (as readers of this book can easily see) are precisely those to which the strongest exception should be taken, which, in a word, should never have taken place at all. But those responsible have gone cheerfully ahead, knowing that they have no

---

[1] Quoted in *Medical News* (London), 10 April 1964.

fear of any objection members of the public might raise, if they were in the habit of reading and could understand the published reports, for the simple reason that the general public will never see these reports and could not understand them if they did. At the same time the experimenters have been able to go ahead equally without any fear that the editors of the medical journals themselves are going to object to an interesting article on some new piece of investigation simply because that particular investigation has offended medical or 'ordinary' ethics. This brings me to the suggestion I wish to make.

If medical editors themselves refused to publish papers which did not furnish evidence that the experiments they reported had been carried out in terms of the principles suggested, then the knowledge that the account of an unjustifiable experiment would not be published would, I believe, give considerable pause to those about to embark on such an experiment. I therefore suggest that this innovation might be made by all medical editors: no reports of experiments to be accepted for publication unless the editor is satisfied that what was done did not offend against any of the principles of medical experiments. This is not, of course, a novel idea. In the memorandum which I have already quoted a very similar recommendation is made:[1]

> A further matter to which the Council would draw attention is that of propriety in publication. It cannot be assumed that it will be evident to every reader that the investigations being described were unobjectionable. Unless such is made unmistakably clear misconceptions can arise. In this connection a special responsibility devolves upon the editors, and editorial boards, of scientific journals. In the Council's opinion, it is desirable that editors and editorial boards, before accepting any communication, should not only satisfy themselves that the appropriate requirements have been fulfilled, but may properly insist that the reader is left in no doubt that such indeed is the case.

The American Professor of Law previously quoted expressed the opinion:

> The possibility of still another safeguard might be a requirement, that all the results of the experiment be submitted to

[1] *Medical Research Memorandum*, 1953/649.

publication, whether they are negative or not, as a check on any overly optimistic, exuberant or ambitious experimenter.[1]

In a previous chapter I have made the suggestion that just as in Great Britain there is published a full official account of all vivisection experiments, so there should be a similar publication listing all experiments on patients, giving the name of the doctor or doctors, the purpose and methods of the experiment (perhaps in brief technical jargon), the complications encountered, and the journal if any in which an account of the experiment has or will be published. I have a strong suspicion that at present both in England and America the most reprehensible experiments are those which are never published either because of unsatisfactory or negative results. This is likely to be especially true of those experimenters who have a passion for being the first to try out some new technique.

[1] F. A. Freund, of Harvard Law School, *New England Journal Medicine*, 1965, **273**, 687.

CONCLUSION

I. REAL VOLUNTEERS

If medical experiments are to be restricted to those which are carried out in conformity with the principles I have suggested, and controlled by legislation in which those principles are embodied, it is obvious that the number of experiments undertaken would be enormously reduced. And while some of this reduction would in no way impede real research (the cessation of experiments made to confirm what is already established, to practise techniques of investigation or to pursue lines of research which are misconceived at the start would be no loss in this respect), there can be no doubt that research itself, in so far as it depends on medical experiment, would be substantially slowed up.

To avoid any such slowing-up is doubtless the motive, or a motive, of many doctors now carrying out experiments which do offend against these principles; their argument is: 'If we took all this into account and only went to work as conscientiously as you are recommending, we would get nowhere with our investigations.' And I have no doubt that this point of view will be advanced as an argument against the recognition of these principles and against their incorporation in law.

But while it is my contention that these principles should be honoured, and research which denies them should be prohibited, even if research itself suffered as a result, I do not think that the second is an inevitable consequence of the first. Many and perhaps all valid experiments which would be fruitful for research could, I believe, still be undertaken under a totally different system. The research-workers could appeal, publicly and openly, for real volunteers. The purpose of the proposed experiment could be plainly announced and the risk involved plainly enunciated. And public-spirited citizens, generous and courageous enough to accept the unpleasantness and the risk, would, I believe, come forward. When approached honestly and directly, most societies turn out to have, among their members, a sufficient number of people willing to risk even their *lives* in a good cause. And a risk of quite that dimension ought not to be necessary here.

215

Conclusion

If this is *not* the case and if volunteers were not forthcoming for a particular experiment, honestly appealed for, then surely the undertaking of that same experiment on uninformed *non*-volunteers, which is what often happens at present, must in consequence be condemned.

Within certain limits I see no objection to paying genuine volunteers, provided that the following suggested safeguards are met.

> Giving of payment may effect the reality of consent. I suggest amounts should not be so large as to constitute undue influance, that is, so large as to obscure the appreciation of the risk and weaken the will to self preservation. We ought not to be put in the business of buying lives.[1]

In some American hospitals agreement of a patient to participate in research is rewarded by a reduction, or complete wavering, of hospital expenses. I do not advocate any extension of this system, because it savours of the exploitation of those economically less well off. This has indeed been recently admitted.[2]

> In so far as clinical research programs were limited to charity patients in the past (that is, prior to the passage of Public Law 89-97 in 1966) these programs may lose some of their 'material'. In our view this is all to the good, as we find a serious dilemma involved in segregating patients for research by their ability to pay for hospital care.

An additional interesting point raised in this article is:

> A problem which has faced clinical investigation in the past is that of paying for the additional tests and procedures. Such additional expenses in the past have been, at least for the most part, covered by research funds rather than by patient care funds. But, as we are all aware, clear distinctions are often difficult to make (that is, between what is research and what is necessary investigation). There may be a temptation to use medical funds to lengthen the patient's stay for research purposes.

[1] Professor F. A. Freund, in Gay Lecture, Harvard Law School, quoted from *New England Journal Medicine*, 1965, **273**, 687.

[2] R. H. Ebert and W. Sidels, of Boston, Mass., *Clinical Research* (Washington), 1966, **14**, 193.

The Return of the Physician-Friend

2. THE RETURN OF THE PHYSICIAN-FRIEND

There would also be a beneficial result, not immediately obvious to the public but of great importance to them – and both obvious and important to the medical profession itself – if real instead of pretended volunteers were used in medical research and if what was really happening in research was consequently out in the open. What I mean concerns the teaching of medicine, the means by which graduates in medicine whose abilities and industry are exceptional may get promotion, and the clinical charge of patients in hospitals.

The first two of these and often the third are intimately connected with the practice of research experiments.

The teachers in our medical schools are often more interested in research and research experiments than in the clinical care of patients. As a result those whom they teach, both under- and post-graduates, are easily infected with the doctrine that what matters first is science and what comes second is the patient. This is the case at some of the highest sources of medical teaching and, as a result, many of the most intelligent young doctors may spend several years after qualification right away from patients and engrossed in back-room techniques.

An equally common result is that a great deal of time is spent by newly qualified doctors working on medical experiments, in order to assemble some original data or perfect some new technique, not necessarily one which is of any real use. These are the means by which, in time, they will be able to submit material to a medical journal and thus gain publication. Through publication the chances of promotion are vastly increased. Having done research and having published papers about it now constitute the royal road to getting on in the medical world. Not only, however, is much of this research ill conceived from the point of view of pure medicine; the pursuit of it has meant the diversion of many a young and often brilliant doctor from that gaining of clinical as opposed to research experience which, in time, could have made him into a considerable physician. But when applying for the post of hospital consultant he has found the state of affairs where those making the appointment have come to regard a grain of research experience as worth a ton of clinical experience. As the

217

doyen of British cardiologists, Sir John Parkinson, said at an International Congress of Cardiology, held at Washington, D.C., in September 1954:

> Must every ambitious graduate be forced by custom or authority to prosecute research in order to obtain a University post or to succeed as a practising cardiologist? Research ability used to be regarded as a rare gift, something of a phenomenon . . . This is not the attitude today . . . My question concerns the universality of the capacity for research; and I almost believe that the true investigator, great or small, is born not made . . . In my view, we encourage good men, inept for research, to sacrifice their time and energy upon it, when they should be perfecting themselves as bedside physicians. Are we losing our sense of proportion, exhilarated by the wonderful products of recent and current research? Is a born investigator a superior being to a born clinician or teacher? He may or may not be. Advances in medicine comprise two separate stages; first the discovery of something new and valuable as the result of investigation; secondly the application of that new discovery to the benefit of the individual patient. The same man may not be the right one for both stages, though he can be. Though commoner than aptitude for research, the power to apply new and old knowledge judiciously is not given to everyone. It also requires a gift – namely clinical judgement. This will ripen to clinical wisdom only by constant association with the sick. Young physicians of this type – so badly wanted – need to keep themselves abreast of world literature in their speciality, and devote time to post-graduate clinical work at other centres and in other lands. Must they invariably be forced to shorten the time required for this large purpose, to participate in minor and often ephemeral research before they are considered for any important staff appointment as a teacher or consultant? Not every young physician should be under compulsion to prosecute individual research in order to succeed.[1]

One of the great present needs of the medical profession is for more general practitioners. The position in Britain is that but for the influx of medical graduates from abroad the National Health Service itself could hardly keep going. Yet the over-emphasized attractions and importance of research continually lead graduates of ability away from this great need into what

[1] *Lancet,* 1955, **1**, 1013, and *Circulation,* 1954.

The Return of the Physician-Friend

Dr. Graef, speaking at a medical conference in New York in 1962, designated a luxury.

> In this era of attention to research, 'glamour', security and academic opportunities offer advantages to the new graduate over the increasing burdens of general practice. The diversion of able physicians to research may become a luxury to the community, where there is a sheer lack of physicians in so many areas of our medical economy.

And what Dr. Graef said about America certainly applies here. Indeed the 'luxury' itself can be a pretty doubtful one from the point of view of the patient, as another American doctor, Dr. Whitehorn, pointed out in an address given in Boston in 1961.

> The technically trained physician, as distinguished from the educated physician, may try impulsively, by the unwise and neurotic multiplication of tests and superfluous instrumentation, to achieve the illusion of certainty, and such behaviour may be only a manifestation of another type of superstition, the superstitious faith in the laboratory report. Such a physician, technically overloaded but inadequately educated in the humane sense, is often constrained to maintain, in the face of his patients, a phony attitude of omniscience, which is likely to evoke in individual patients an uneasy suspicion and distrust.

The maintenance of a 'phony attitude of omniscience' is a very sorry activity for a doctor and is one of the several results of putting second things first which it has been the aim of this book to point out. As a great physician, the late Sir Robert Hutchinson, put the matter:

> From inability to let well alone, from too much zeal for the new, and contempt for what is old; from putting knowledge before wisdom, science before art, cleverness before common sense; from treating patients as cases; and from making 'the cure' of the disease more grievous than the endurance of the same, Good Lord deliver us.[1]

[1] *British Medical Journal*, 1953, 1, 671.

INDEX

Eichna, 120, 122
Eisenmenger, 136
Eithelberger, 61
Elithorn, A., 39
Emmanoulides, 40, 41
Engel, F. L., 106
Epstein, R. M., 90
Espit, M., 56
Estes, 105
Evans, A. S., 83

Farber, S. J., 122
Faris, 66
Farrar, Betty, 131
Fazekas, 54, 145
Fazell, 72
Feinberg, 54
Felson, 73
Ferguson-Smith, 58
Ferrer, Irene, 154
Figley, M. M., 24, 69
Filler, 91
Finlayson, J. K., 156
Finnerty, F. A., 147
Fisher, Arthur, 70
Fisher, D. A., 99
Fisher, R. E. W., 32, 58
Fishman, A. P., 90
Fishman, R. A., 59
Fitzpatrick, H. F., 88
Foman, S. J., 46
Foot, E. C., 168
Forman, Harris, 119
Foster, J. H., 23
Fox, R. C., 4, 61
Fox, Wayne, 126
Fraser, Russel, 103
Freeman, M., 110
Freeman, N. E., 72
Freidberg, S. J., 105
Freund, F. A., 7, 32, 67, 125, 202, 212, 216
Frische, 14
Fries, 116

Frumin, M. J., 90
Fry, W. J., 69
Frye, R. L., 144

Gabe, I., 153, 163
Gabuzda, 116
Garrard, 32
Gasul, 37
Geronimo, 181
Gilfillian, 72
Gleeson, J. A., 171
Gloster, Josephine, 151, 152
Glover, W. E., 85
Glynn, L. E., 39
Goldberg, Harry, 158
Goldberg, L. I., 169
Goldfinch, 32
Goldring, 90
Goluboff, 57
Goodwin, W. E., 13
Gordon, E. E., 113
Gorezyea, 107
Gorlin, R., 120, 121
Graber, 87
Graef, 219
Graettinger, 153
Grainger, R. G., 24
Grant, D. Kerr, 74
Grauaug, 37
Gray, R. E., 37
Greene, M. A., 179
Gregory, R., 142
Greenfield, A. D. M., 85
Groote, de, 134, 136
Grossman, L., 39
Guervera, 108
Guillaudeu, 147
Gurtner, 177
Guthrie, J., 168
Guttentag, O. E., 10, 11, 78, 196
Guy, Laren, 182

Habif, D. V., 88, 90
Hackel, D. B., 145

Index